HEALTHY FOOD

~For Diabetes, Celiac Disease and You!~

Sharon Fox

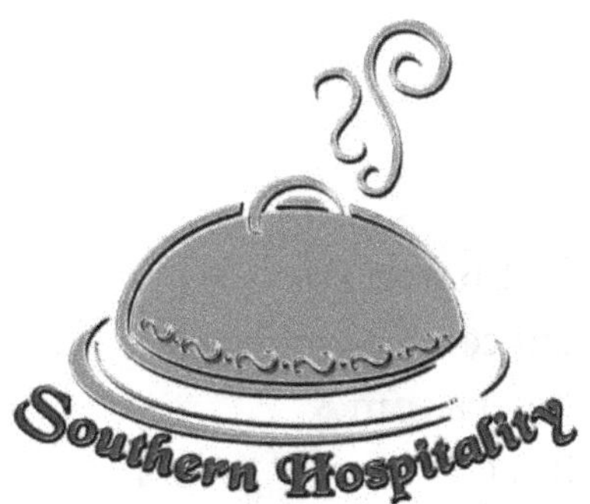

Southern Hospitality Books, LLC

Cover designed by: Donna Osborn Clark at:
CreationsbyDonna@gmail.com
Interior designed by: Glenda Wallace at: interiorbookdesigns.com

ISBN: 0615720153
ISBN-13: 978-0615720159

Contact information for Sharon Fox:
goodcooking4u2@gmail.com
www.goodcookin4u2.webs.com
facebook.com/ icook4real
twitter.com/ ImSharonFox

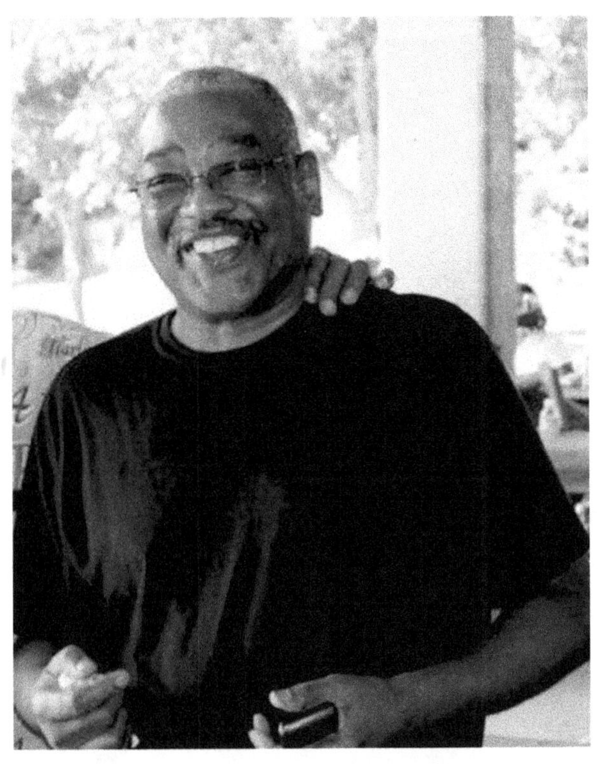

I dedicate this work to my father, Garner Ray Skelton. He was always the driving force I needed to pursue my career in writing and helping enrich the lives of others.

Rest in peace Daddy, I will always love you.

5/26/1945 - 2/8/2012

Acknowledgments

Thanks to everyone who encouraged me to write this book:
Robert and Pamela Coleman
Ryan Walker
Eugene Williams
Donna Osborn Clark
Ricky Aaron
Carol Trainer
and especially my sons Bryant, Brandon, Bradley, and Jaalan.
Special love for my grand children Exodus and Triniti (due in January 2013)
I pray that many lives will be enriched by the dedication I had in putting all of this hard work and research together. Live your best life, take care of your Self, and love one another!

Contents

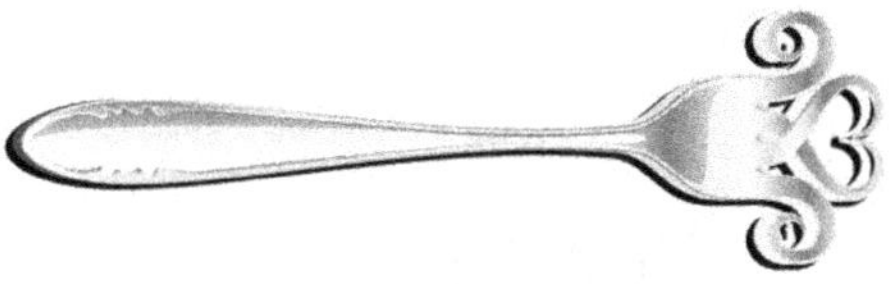

Chapter 1

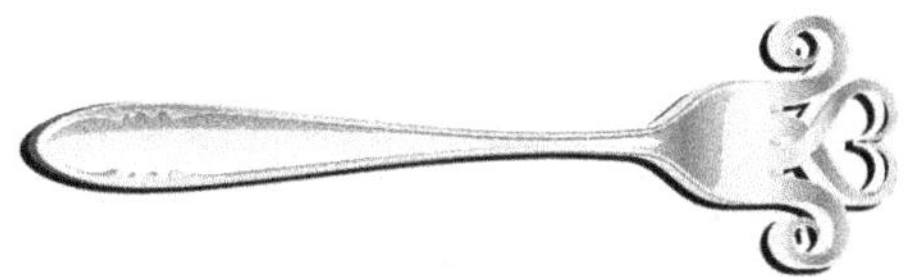

~THE DIABETES LIFESTYLE~

I heard a dear friend say, "If you want to get scared into good health, get diagnosed with Diabetes. " This disease will literally force you into examining your eating and exercise habits and will tune you into your body's signal and response system. You must be required to commit to regular preventative care and for some people it's a great motivation for positive health changes like losing weight and giving up smoking.

Good diabetes management must also become a lifestyle choice. Simple tasks like eating a good meal, going for a walk or bicycle ride, and going on a weekend trip will take extra preparation and planning. Your daily routines like working and going to school begin to pose new challenges, and special occasions sometimes seem particularly hard to deal with. Even the change of seasons can mean changes in your diabetes control. As if that's not enough, age and gender can make good control a challenge of its own - children, adults, and the elderly all face unique treatment needs and trials.

It's not surprising that many people living with Diabetes also face emotional and psychological issues such as depression and denial. Coping with the daily demands of any chronic disease can be hard and often discouraging. The great news is that the hard work pays off. Even minor lifestyle improvements such as adding 30 minutes of exercise to your daily routine can pay off big by lowering your blood glucose levels and significantly cutting your risk of diabetic complications.

The Smallest Patients: Babies and Toddlers

If you are a parent, then you definitely know that not knowing how to help your hurting child is a horrible feeling. When little ones have Diabetes, they can't tell you if they are "feeling low " or need to check their blood glucose. We as parents learn the difference between a "wet cry " and a "hungry cry " and parents of Diabetic children become attuned to the signs of their child's feelings as well.

Recognizing the Signs and Symptoms

The very same symptoms that older children and adults have signaling the possibility of Type 1 Diabetes also apply to babies and toddlers; the difference being that verbal communication is limited, so you probably won't recognize them as quickly. Symptoms like fatigue are hard to detect in a baby who sleeps a great deal of the day anyway. Most parents will take a "better safe than sorry " attitude and take the inconsolable infant or toddler to the doctor to find out what's wrong rather than waiting around to see if the issue goes away. This is the best move to make in any case. If the child is not acting "normal ", always get a doctor to check him/her out. If your child is at risk of Type 1 Diabetes, you can watch out for these symptoms:

- Excessive wet diapers
- Diaper rash that doesn't heal quickly, or keeps recurring
- Constant hunger/thirst
- Irritability or fussiness not related to colic
- Sleeping more than usual

Noticing the Highs and Lows

Recognizing the blood sugar highs and lows may be very complicated when Diabetes has been diagnosed in a very young child. The best tool for making sure things are in balance is a glucose monitor. If the child is acting abnormal, always check the glucose levels first. It may not be the Diabetes, but if it is you want to find out as quickly as possible and treat it fast. Talk to your child's doctor about the appropriate amount of carbohydrates to treat the "lows ". As a general rule, children under the age of six require 5 to 10 grams of fast-acting carb for each 50mg/ dl blood glucose is low.

Medi-Tip:

If you have a baby or toddler with Diabetes, keep an oral syringe handy to administer a fast acting carb like syrup if a hypo occurs and the baby refuses a bottle of juice. Cake frosting in a tube and glucose gel can also work for more cooperative eaters. Never feed a child who has lost consciousness because of the risk of choking, and NEVER give an infant a glucose tablet or hard candy.

Monitoring Glucose

Glucose checks can be a complicated task for parents, especially in very young children who don't understand why they must be poked. You can make your job easier by purchasing an alternate site meter, which allows you to test on less sensitive areas like the forearm. You may also stick the heel of the foot instead of the fingers. Always talk to your doctor for recommendations. Just remember, your child will eventually get used to the checks.

Insulin and Eating

Little ones are known for having unpredictable appetites. They can go for days eating very little, and then suddenly eat a whole plate of spaghetti and meatballs like a big boy or girl. The problem is, you never know what your child is going to gobble up or push away at the next meal, so this makes giving insulin a bit difficult. This is the reason your doctor may recommend short-acting insulin to be administered immediately after a meal to cover the carbs and avoid highs or lows.

Insulin injections can be really hard for a child, but there are many injection aids on the market to make the job a lot easier on both of you. Your doctor can prescribe a topical anesthetic cream to numb the injection site. There is also a device called an Inject-Ease that can be used with a standard syringe to both hide the needle and minimize pain by facilitating a rapid injection. You can also try simple home methods like numbing the area with ice, a frozen treat, or cold water bottle.

Help Your Child Manage Diabetes

You know your child better than anyone, so use that knowledge to gradually introduce him to the different aspects of self-management at the appropriate time. Remember that all children mature at different rates; what one child can handle at age seven another may be ready for at age four. Each child's emotional and physical development can also progress at different rates. For this reason, a pre-school child may have the mental capacity to test his own blood glucose levels, but lack fine motor skills to do the job. However, the smallest child can be empowered to take part in his Diabetes care by reading a blood glucose monitor screen, unzipping a supply case, or choosing an injection or testing site. Here are a few basic Diabetes management skills and general guidelines on when your child may be able to take them on:

- **Self-testing blood sugar levels.** Between ages 5 and 7 children may start expressing an interest in testing their own blood glucose levels. As long as their testing method is correct, there is no reason not to pass along this little task to your child. By age 8 most children can master this task (unless they are newly diagnosed). As a parent, you must remind the child to test at the appropriate times and help interpret blood sugar readings.

- **Counting the Carbs.** Between ages 7 and 9 the child may ask about carbohydrates and engage in basic carb counting. Children's educational systems that use visual aids such as flash cards or refrigerator magnets may help your child understand carb counting at an early age.

- **Taking Insulin.** Between ages 8 and 12 most children should be able to administer their injections; of course parents should always oversee the dose calculation and drawing up of the insulin, although doing so in a hands off manner will help your child build the skills and confidence needed to take over this task himself. The same goes for regulating the insulin pump therapy.

Teens Managing Diabetes

There are unique issues for teens facing Diabetes. Simple things like going to birthday parties, playing sports, or going on a trip with friends need careful planning. Everyday children with Diabetes may need to take insulin or oral medications. They also need to remember to check their blood glucose several times a day and remember to eat the right foods. These tasks can make them feel different from their other friends and classmates and can be particularly bothersome for teens.

Dealing with a chronic disease like Diabetes may cause emotional or behavioral challenges. Talking to a social worker or psychologist may help you and your teen adjust to lifestyle changes needed to stay healthy. Managing Diabetes in teens is most effective when the entire family makes a team effort. Share your concerns with doctors, dietitians and other health care professionals to get the very best information and care for your child. These individuals may also be able to help with resources for health education, financial services, social services, mental health counseling, transportation, and home visiting. Diabetes can be very stressful for both teens and their families. Parents should always be alert for signs of depression or eating disorders in order to seek the appropriate treatment. All parents should talk to their children about avoiding tobacco. People with Diabetes who smoke have a considerably higher risk of heart disease and circulatory problems. Binge drinking can increase the risk of low blood sugar (hypoglycemia) and the symptoms can easily be mistaken for those of intoxication and not properly treated. Local peer groups for children and teens with Diabetes can provide positive role models and group activities.

Diabetes and Women

According to the American Diabetes Association, an estimated 11.5 million women over age 20 in the United States have Diabetes. Did you know that over one-third of them remain undiagnosed? In comparison to men, women have a 50 percent greater risk of diabetic coma. This is a condition brought on by poorly controlled Diabetes and lack of insulin. Women with Diabetes have heart disease rates similar to men, but more women with Diabetes die from their first heart attack.

Diabetic Complications and Women

- Cardiovascular Disease. This is the most common complication attributable to Diabetes, and is more serious among women than men. Death from heart disease in women with Diabetes have increased 23% over the past 30 years, compared to a 27% decrease in women without Diabetes.

- ❖ Peripheral Vascular Disease (PVD). Women with Diabetes are 7.6 times as likely to suffer PVD than women without Diabetes. PVD is a disorder resulting in reduced flow of blood and oxygen to tissues in the feet and legs. The main symptom of PVD is pain in the thigh, calf, or buttocks during exercise.
- ❖ Diabetic Ketoacidosis (DKA). The risk of DKA is 50% higher among women than men. DKA is often called Diabetic coma and is brought on by poorly controlled Diabetes and marked by high blood glucose levels. DKA is not caused by high blood sugar, but by lack of insulin. Before insulin therapy was available, DKA was the predominant cause of death from Diabetes.

Women of Color and Diabetes

Diabetes is one of the most serious health problems facing women in the United States today, especially women of color. Complications from this disease rank among the top 10 causes of death for all women, especially women of color.

Among African American women, type 2 Diabetes has reached epidemic proportions; 11.8% for those age 20 or over.

Almost 1 in 4 black women over the age of 55 has Diabetes, nearly twice the rate of white women.

25% of Latina women have been diagnosed with type 2 Diabetes, and about 33% of deaths among them list Diabetes as the underlying cause. This rate has risen sharply in the past 30 years.

American Indian/Alaskan Native women have almost 3 times the risk of being diagnosed with Diabetes as whites of similar age. This disease is common in many tribes and the sickness and mortality can be very severe.

Older American Indian/Alaskan Native and Mexican American women are among the most likely to have Diabetes. (32% American Indian/Alaskan Native, 30% Mexican American, 25% African American, and 15% White women). Diabetes-related health risks are two-fold: health risks that can lead to Diabetes and health risks that result from having Diabetes. The risks associated with having this disease are: loss of vision and blindness, foot ulcers, lower extremity amputations, and pregnancy and cardiovascular complications. In addition, Diabetes is associated with birth defects, high blood pressure, nervous system damage, dental disease, stroke, and flu and pneumonia-related deaths.

Cardiovascular disease is the most costly complication of Diabetes, accounting for almost $20 billion in health costs annually- and rising. African Americans experience higher rates of Diabetic complications such as eye disease, kidney failure, amputations, and heart disease.

Diabetes and Men

Men with Diabetes suffer more from some diabetes-related health problems than women. The American diabetes Association reported that:

Before age 30, men develop retinopathy (a vision disorder that can lead to blindness) more quickly than women.

Having the main symptoms of PVD (peripheral vascular disease), cramps, sores that won't heal, or swelling. This is linked to the increased risk of coronary heart disease, stroke, or cardiac failure in men with Diabetes.

Amputation rates from Diabetes-related problems are 2 to 2.5 times higher in men than women with Diabetes.

Erectile Dysfunction

Erectile Dysfunction is not uncommon in men with Diabetes. A diagnosis will be made by your doctor:

- Patient History: Medical and sexual histories will help define the degree and nature of ED. Your medical history can disclose issues that led to the dysfunction, while a simple recounting of sexual activity might distinguish among problems with sexual desire, erection, ejaculation, and orgasm. Certain drugs, whether prescription or illegal, have been accountable for over 25% of ED cases. Your doctor will be able to tell you if a certain drug is the problem or if it's actually Diabetes.

- Physical Exam: An examination can give clues to systemic problems. For example, if the penis is not sensitive to touching, a problem with the nervous system may be the cause. Abnormal secondary sex characteristics such as hair pattern or breast enlargement may point to hormonal problems. The doctor may even discover a circulatory problem by checking pulse points of the wrist or ankles. Unusual characteristics of the penis itself, like bending or curving while erect, may suggest the source of the problem.

- Lab Tests: There are many lab tests that can be done to help diagnose ED. Blood counts, urinalysis, lipid profile, and measurements of liver enzymes are just a few. Measuring the amount of testosterone in the blood will give your doctor information about the endocrine system, especially in patients with decreased sexual desire.

- There are many other tests that may be done to diagnose the ED problem. The sexual partner may even be asked to complete a questionnaire to help the doctor evaluate the issue. Just remember that there are many solutions to ED for Diabetics. Just be completely open with your doctor, your partner, and yourself so that your solution can possibly be resolved. Diabetes can create several issues in your life, but once you are comfortable discussing all the problems with your doctor, the life of a Diabetic can get easier by the day. Remember that you are not the only person to ever have these problems, and you will learn how to handle your own personal issues with the help of your doctors and support of your loved ones. Your life is not over, it's only just begun. There is a whole new way of living that is designed especially for you. Enjoy every moment of it. Take care of yourself to the best of your ability and be grateful for every moment you have to make new memories!

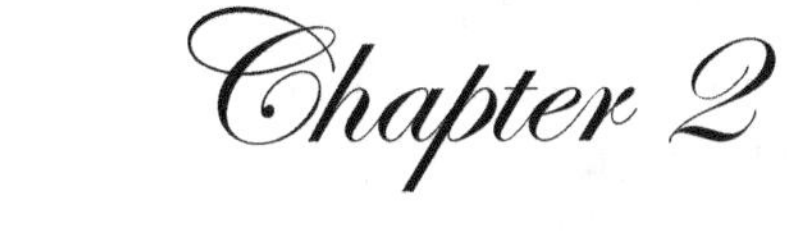

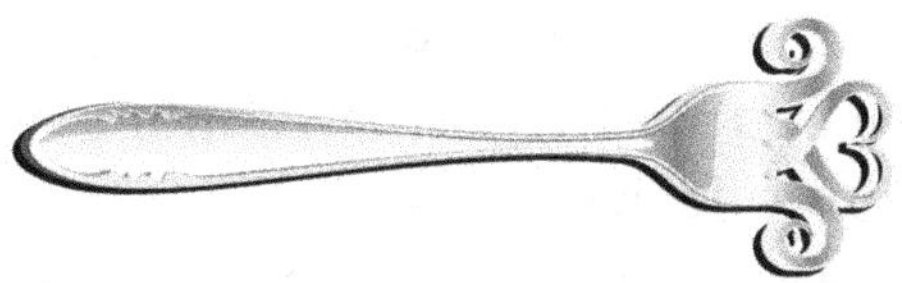

~WEIGHT CONTROL~

Controlling the weight is one of the top issues for many people living with type 2 Diabetes. Being overweight is a risk factor for developing Diabetes and also promotes insulin resistance. Too much body fat makes it harder for the body to use the insulin it makes to process blood glucose. Because excess blood sugar is stored by the body as fat, uncontrolled Diabetes can make weight control even more difficult.

Top Weight Loss Tips

- **Use that measuring tape!** When it comes to shedding body fat, the scale is not always your friend. The very best way to slim down is to simultaneously change your eating habits and increase physical activity. Remember this: Exercising builds muscle mass, which is a good thing for you. So, if you seriously increase your weight-bearing exercise, your weight could actually go up. This is because muscle tissue is more metabolically active than other body tissue, so the more muscle you have, the more calories your body burns while you rest. Muscle weighs more than fat. The measuring tape won't lie. As you lose body fat, you lose inches around your waist, hips, thighs, and upper arms. Eventually you won't even need the tape. Your jeans will tell you all you need to know!

❖ **Indulge in Soup!** Have you noticed how full you feel after a good bowl of soup? This is a great weight-loss secret. A bowl of broth-based soup with veggies and beans (try kale, onions, and white beans in chicken broth) can be a terrific strategy for weight loss. Make a habit of having a bowl of soup for lunch or dinner every day, adding a whole grain to it every other day. Make it yourself because canned soups can be packed with sodium.

❖ **Learn from Former Smokers!** Changing your eating habits can be a lot like quitting smoking. You'll need to learn to dodge those cravings instead of indulging in them. When you are tempted by that pasta dish or decadent dessert, try the craving busters that smokers use:

1. Count to 30, slowly. The craving will slowly subside. You may have to do it more than once.
2. Visualize a thinner you. Meditate on what you want to look like and know that you deserve to be thinner and healthier. When you focus on the end result, it will help you control your desire to indulge.
3. Find a new habit like drinking some green tea, taking a walk, or crunching on some celery or piece of fruit.
4. Change your routine. Do some stretches while watching your favorite TV show instead of having a bag of chips. Call a friend and chit chat for awhile. Do a puzzle or take up a craft to keep your hands busy.
5. Just say NO! If you really must eat something, make it healthy. Don't allow your cravings to take control over you. You must stay in control at all times.

- **Make Mental Notes!** Without realizing it, you may use food as a comfort, distraction, pleaser, or stress reliever. If you feel that you use food for these reasons, consult your doctor for help with this issue. Using food as an answer to psychological issues is very common and can be cured.

- **Change it up!** Instead of thinking about all the foods you must avoid, celebrate all the new foods that you can add to shake up your meal plans. Try a new whole grain, fruit, or vegetable each week. Experiment with new fruits, vegetables, kasha, spaghetti squash, or papaya. Keep a list of your favorites and use them in some of your favorite recipes.

- **Invest your time!** This is a great tip for anyone trying to lose weight, but especially for those who eat too fast. Try foods that take some time to eat. Foods that slow you down like kiwi, crab, or even a hard-boiled egg. If you have to work to get to the good stuff, you won't take in as many calories.

- **Re-train your taste buds!** It is a proven fact that when people give up salt, even lightly-salted foods begin to taste terribly salty. The same is true for people who give up sugar- things start tasting really sweet. Try to decrease your salt and sugar intake. Also extend this concept to foods made with white flour. If you eliminate certain things from your diet, the cravings for these items disappear as well!

- **Drink water!** If you drink 1-2 glasses of water before you eat, it will cause you to consume fewer calories. It's even better if the water is cold. Your digestive system has to burn energy to warm the water in your body, thus burning even more calories.

Diabetic Diet?

One thing I truly get annoyed by is when people talk about the "Diabetic Diet". In my opinion, there is no such thing. Diabetes is not a "life sentence" to a rigid meal plan or special diet that deprives your from all the foods you love. This is mostly myth. The eating habits or "diet" for a person with Diabetes is actually the same healthy diet that's best for everyone! If we all ate like the doctors suggest for Diabetics, there would virtually be no such thing as Diabetes.

We all need to limit sugars, control carbs, eat plenty of fruits and vegetables, and exercise regularly. I suggest to everyone to honestly make an effort to treat their bodies with love, honor, and respect. We were all given a life, and it is up to us to take care of it. Before you put anything in your mouth, think about the affects it will have on the only body you have. If you continue to eat this "thing" regularly, how will it make your body feel over time?

It's normal to treat yourself to something special now and then, but don't kill yourself by going overboard. If you are Diabetic, respect your illness and program your mind to knowing that YOU are in control...your disease is not. Care for your body in a way that Diabetes cannot kill you if you don't allow it to do so. Eat to live, don't live to eat! You should want to enjoy every moment of everyday of your life. We all need food to sustain our bodies, but we must not let unhealthy foods control our lives to the point of destroying us.

Chapter 3

~SUGARS, CARBS, AND FATS~

Let's take a look at how carbohydrates work. When we eat, the carbohydrates in our food become glucose in our blood. Certain foods are higher in carbs - potatoes and pasta, sugar, bread and cereal - and they cause blood glucose levels to spike. People with Diabetes have to manage their intake of carbs to avoid these spikes. Carb counting and after- meal blood sugar testing are the best ways to determine your daily carbohydrate intake. You don't have to be a Diabetic to eat like one. Actually, if we all watched our sugars, pastas, and carbohydrate-rich food intake, we'd all be a lot healthier. This chapter will shed some light on the true facts about the main things that affect your blood glucose. There are many questions that may be in the back of your mind that I hope to answer for you. What are carbs? Are there "good" carbs and "bad" carbs? How can a potato be in the same category as a slice of cake? Let's move on and get right to it.

Sugars and Artificial Sweeteners

With most foods and drinks, the sweeter it is, the higher the carb count is. That is exactly why it's so important to understand the ups and downs of naturally occurring sugars, added sugars, and artificial sweeteners. ***Naturally occurring sugars*** exist in fruits, vegetables, and all dairy products. Did you know that ***lactose*** is a sugar? ***Added sugars*** would be table sugar, cane sugar, corn syrup, evaporated cane juice, molasses, and the like. Finally, ***artificial sweeteners.*** They are nonnutritive, they have no nutritional value at all. They are low in calories and carbs. The most popular names are aspartame, saccharine, and sucralose. You are familiar with the little pink, blue, or yellow packets on the counters of your favorite coffee shops or on the table at your local restaurants. Knowing a little about how foods and drinks are sweetened will give you a head start on making wise decisions on what will fit into your personal healthy eating plans and what doesn't.

Sugar Substitutes: The Scoop

There is a myth that Diabetics can't eat any sugar. But Diabetics can have foods and drinks sweetened with sugar if you work them into a smart eating plan, taking your carbohydrates into account. Having too many sweets can push your blood sugar out of the target range, this is why sugar substitutes can be used to satisfy that sweet tooth while allowing you to maintain control. There are two types of sugar substitutes available on the market today - non-calorie and reduced-calorie sweeteners.

Non-calorie Sweeteners.

These artificial sweeteners contain no calories, no carbohydrates, and do not raise blood sugar levels. They can be used to sweeten drinks, desserts, and candies. Some can even be used in cooking and baking. Some of the most popular brands are: NutraSweet, Equal, Sweet'N Low, and Splenda. As stated earlier, these artificial sweeteners do not raise blood sugar. If your blood sugar jumps after you eat an artificially sweetened food, the culprit may be other ingredients in the food such as caffeine, carbohydrates, or protein. Even stress can spike your blood sugar.

Reduced-calorie Sweeteners.

These are also known as ***sugar alcohols***, even though they don't contain any alcohol at all! They are made by chemically altering natural sugar and metabolized very differently. These artificial sweeteners DO contain carbohydrates and some calories, although less than real sugar. They are commonly found in packaged foods like cookies, candy, and gum. Common names for these sweeteners are: sorbitol, mannitol, lactitiol, maltitol, xylitol, isomalt, erythritol, and hydrogenated starch hydrolysates.

These products DO raise blood sugar. The American Diabetes Association recommends subtracting half of the sugar alcohol grams when computing a food's total carb count. For example, if a store bought cereal bar contains6 grams of sugar alcohol and a total of 15 grams of carbohydrates, you'd count it as 12 grams of carbohydrates (15-3=12).

Are these artificial sweeteners safe?

Although the FDA considers artificial sweeteners safe, saccharin was believed to cause bladder cancer in the past. Further research determined that it posed no danger to humans. Aspartame has been accused of causing headaches, although there are no reliable studies to support this claim.

As with any food, moderation is the best policy if you decide that artificial sweeteners are your sugar of choice. Just remember, foods that are high in artificial sweeteners leave less room for fresh vegetables, whole grains, protein-rich foods, and fresh fruit. It's always best to get your sugars from nature. I'd personally suggest that you get more of what God created and less of what was manufactured to temporarily satisfy a sweet tooth.

Remember, if you get hooked on sweetening everything, you'll never get used to eating things unsweetened or in its natural state. Try to slowly push away from artificial sweeteners and enjoy the foods that nature gives you.

Everyone can't eat artificial sweeteners anyway. Some people have trouble tolerating them. Sugar alcohols can cause bloating, flatulence, or diarrhea.

If you decide to use artificial sweeteners or eat those products, please keep in mind that labels can be misleading. Just because a label claims that an item is "sugar-free" doesn't necessarily mean it's calorie-free or carbohydrate-free. They may still have significant amounts of carbs and calories either because they are sweetened with sugar alcohols or other non-sugar sweeteners or because they contain other high-carbohydrate ingredients. Always pay close attention to the total carbohydrate content listed on the food labels.

Artificial Sweetener Alternatives.

There are natural sweeteners that you may find quite satisfying and more tolerable, and definitely healthier for you. As with any sweetener, you still need to use them in moderation. As I stated before, try to eat what nature provides. Here are some healthy choices:

- **Agave Nectar:** This natural sweetener comes from the agave plant. It is much sweeter than sugar, so a little goes a long way. Many people find it has a lower impact on blood sugars as other sweeteners. It does contain carbohydrates, so test vigilantly afterwards until you get used to using it.

- **Stevia:** This is a natural herb that doesn't raise blood sugar levels at all.. The USFDA has found this product very safe, so now you can find it readily available in grocery stores as a sweetener. This is actually my preference, but you definitely have to choose what's best for you.

- **Natural Flavorings:** Believe it or not, very small amounts of vanilla extract, almond extract, lemon, lime, or cinnamon can add flavor to unsweetened foods and give the impression of sweetness! Not a lot, just a touch. "A dab will do ya".

High Fructose Corn Syrup: The Good, the Bad, and the Ugly

You have read or heard about this product in the news, on commercials, and all over the web. Some say it's good for you, some say it's bad. You can make your decision, but I want to share with you my research.

It's sweeter than sugar and cheap! For this reason food and beverage manufacturers use it in almost everything they make including soft drinks, fruit drinks, jams, crackers, bread, yogurt, salad dressing, and even soup! Some researchers stated that fructose is not metabolized in the same way other sugars are, and many experts believe it is no worse than any other sweetener.

Evil Sweetness

In the American Journal of Clinical Nutrition, there was an article published (2004) concluding that there is a distinct likelihood that increased consumption of High Fructose Corn Syrup (HFCS) in beverages may be linked to the increase in obesity. Fructose does NOT stimulate the pancreas to release insulin and does not trigger the secretion of the hormone leptin, which is instrumental in making us feel satisfied. This research also points to the fact that increased use of HFCS is the cause of increased obesity rate in America. HFCS is now used in over

40% of the caloric sweeteners added to foods and drinks produced in the United States.

Corn Refiners Association debunked these statements (of course), stating that HFCS is not actually "high" in fructose. They say it's only 55% fructose and the rest is mostly glucose. They say the proportions are equivalent to table sugar, which is 50% fructose, and 50% glucose. There are articles in magazines both supporting and debunking the facts about HFCS, but in my personal opinion, HFCS should be avoided as much as possible. Any product that has been chemically altered to put in your food raises many questions. If you have to conduct research about something you eat regularly, I don't think you need to eat it.

Fructose and Diabetes

At first glance, one may think eating fructose may alter blood sugar and insulin would "fix" it. Well it's not that simple. First of all fructose is combined with glucose and other sugars to make High Fructose Corn Syrup. Secondly, in animal studies rats were fed large amounts of fructose and became insulin resistant, a precursor to Diabetes. They also developed high triglycerides. Combine this info with the fact that fructose may suppress the release of the appetite-regulating hormone leptin and you have the cocktail for creating obesity. In other words, HFCS stops the necessary hormone needed to make you know that you are full! If you don't feel full, you continue to eat...thus obesity has started.

Whether it's table sugar, honey, or a highly processed sweetener like HFCS, added sugar is something we are better off without-- no matter what your health status is! Get your sugars from natural, healthy sources and you can't go wrong.

All About Fats

There is so many myths and lots of confusion when it comes to fat. The word "fat" represents three totally different things: the soft, squishy stuff that develops around your middle section (body fat), the substance that clogs your arteries (blood fats/cholesterol), and the ingredient we use for cooking (dietary fat). Over the years, dietary fat has come in and out of fashion. For a long time we were taught that fat makes you fat! Today we know better, so we can do better. Moderate amounts of fat found in plants and animals are healthy and even necessary in a nutritionally complete diet. We also know that manufactured fats like hydrogenated oils, also known as trans fats, found in things like crackers and cakes, processed foods, and frozen dinner entrees, are not good for you and have no place in a healthy diet.

Here's the Skinny on Fats

We used to go by our instincts to avoid "fattening" foods. We cut out deep fried foods, rich cakes and pies, and very starchy and cheesy foods because they were all known to be the foods that caused obesity. But after scientists kept probing to find out how diets affect health, things became more confusing. Today most people know that saturated fat has been linked to higher levels of LDL (bad) cholesterol, and linked to be an increased risk for heart disease. Diabetics are automatically in a higher risk group when it comes to heart disease , so most must watch their saturated fat intake. Taught to skip the butter, limiting red meat and cheeses, and using skim milk was the norm. Research has revealed so many facts now that actually pull the curtain off all the myths.

Bad Fats

Trans fats are the worst offenders of all fats. Most manufacturers have lowered and even dropped the use of these fats in their products because of the health risks. Be sure to look closely at ingredient labels to avoid the trans fats in your diet.

Good Fats

In the past 10 years or so, research has repeatedly shown that the healthy fats in fish, olives, nuts, seeds, and avocados deliver potent disease-fighting nutrients. The American Heart Association and American Diabetes Association now recommend that most people eat fish 2-3 times a week. The best choices are salmon, sardines, mackerel, herring, albacore tuna, and rainbow trout. If you have elevated triglycerides or have cardiovascular disease, you may benefit from eating a little more. Talk to your doctor about this and supplementing with fish oil capsules. Fish contains two types of omega-3 fats (EPA and DHA) that have shown to help prevent heart attacks and strokes. Another type of omega-3 fat (ALA) is found in flaxseed, walnuts, canola oil, soybeans, and dark leafy greens. These are extremely heart-healthy foods.

Proportion

Some of our diet-related health problems stem from an imbalance of omega-6 and omega-3 fats. We get omega-6 fats from vegetable oils and omega-3 fats mostly from fish. Today in the American diet, we consume these types of fats at a 10 to 1 ratio, with our consumption of vegetable oils far out-weighing our fish oils. Here are a few tips to help improve your ratio and health:

❖ Eat a variety of (non-fried) fatty fish and seafood 2-3 times a week. If you don't like fish, talk to your doctor about fish oil capsules. You can also look for foods enriched with omega-3 such as eggs and margarines.

❖ Eat a larger variety of plant foods such as nuts, seeds, avocados, olives, and soy foods.

❖ Add ground flaxseed or flaxseed oil, walnuts, and dark green leafy veggies to your rotation each week.

❖ Limit your intake of "junk" foods and processed foods.

❖ Experiment with different foods in this section. You can create salads, add them to your meals, and even begin to substitute some of these items to what you normally eat. Variety is the spice of life! Live your life to the fullest and enjoy every moment of the journey. Nature has given you so many amazing foods. Take a little time to enjoy them.

Chapter 4

~COOKING OILS & SUPER FOODS~

Dietary fat has come in and out of fashion for Diabetics. Before insulin, fat was the primary source of calories of the Diabetic diet. The pendulum swung in the other direction in recent decades, and fat became the dietary villain. Today, fats still reign at the top of the Diabetic Food Pyramid as the food group that should be limited most!

Many researchers argue that with Diabetes, limiting carbs is more important than limiting fat, However, in recent years the pendulum seems to be moving again, with a new emphasis on consuming a variety of natural fats, avoiding the unnatural ones. As I said before, eat what nature has given you!

Trans fats are man-made, so avoid them at all costs. Since 2 out of 3 Diabetics die from heart attack or stroke, it is very important that they choose oils that support a healthy heart.- this means oils that are high in mono and poly-unsaturated fat.

Monounsaturated fats actually help lower the total LDL (bad) cholesterol levels without the negative effect on HDL (good) cholesterol.

Polyunsaturated fats also help lower total cholesterol, but may also lower the good cholesterol in the process. Some poly-unsaturated fats are also good sources of omega-3 fatty acids which are known to decrease the risk of blood clotting and inflammation to help lower the risk of heart disease and has also been linked to lowering the risk of type 1 diabetes.

Knowing which oils are the healthiest is only half the battle. Pairing the right oil with the proper cooking method is important as well. Some oils are good for high heat, while others are best for salad dressings. I have made it a little easier so that you don't have to guess or use a "trial and error" method to discover which is which.

The 10 Best Oils for Diabetics

1. **Walnut Oil:** A polyunsaturated fat and good source for omega-3. This oil is good for baking and to saute at low to medium-high heat. Also good drizzled on salad.
2. **Flaxseed Oil:** A polyunsaturated fat and good source of omega-3. Due to the low smoking point, it's not recommended for cooking over heat. Best for salads.
3. **Canola Oil:** A monounsaturated fat. Great used in baking stir-frying, sauteing, and salad dressings.
4. **Olive Oil:** A monounsaturated fat used as a flavorful oil in sauteing, in sauces, and salad dressings.
5. **Peanut Oil:** A monounsaturated fat. Good for sauteing, sauces, frying, and even salad dressings.
6. **Almond Oil:** A monounsaturated fat. This is a good oil for high heat cooking like frying or sauteing. Very light in taste, so it's good in desserts.
7. **Avocado Oil:** A monounsaturated fat. Good for high heat cooking like frying or sauteing. Tasty in salads as well.
8. **Safflower Oil:** A polyunsaturated fat with a low saturated fatl level.. This makes a good all-purpose oil. Wonderful in high-heat cooking.
9. **Sunflower Oil:** A polyunsaturated fat with a low saturated fat level. Especially good for high heat cooking like frying or sauteing.

10. **Grapeseed Oil:** A polyunsaturated fat with a low saturated fat level. This is a great oil for grilling, frying, stir-frying, and sauteing. The light, nutty flavor also makes it good for salads.

This list is sure to be of assistance in helping you choose the right oil for you.

Now, on to the good stuff. I mentioned to you so many times thus far, to choose foods that nature has supplied. We were always taught from our earliest childhood memories that fruits and veggies are good for us. Needless to say, that is so true. Not just for the nutritional value, but there are so many other health benefits that you may not even be aware of. I want you to take notes on this section. You may want to incorporate more of these foods into your weekly rotation, especially if you have the need to prevent certain illnesses or want to feel better in certain areas of your body.

Some foods have "star power" when it comes to Diabetes. Nature's bounty comes complete with healing nutrients, blood sugar moderating compounds, things that fight cancer, heart disease, and many of the complications that come with Diabetes. Not only do these foods offer healing and healthy benefits, they are all lowest in carbohydrates of all veggies! So remember to pick up some of these items on your next trip to the produce section of your local grocery store. Don't stop until you've tried them all. You'll feel so good offering these items to your loved ones.

ARUGULA contains 2g of carbs in a 50 gram portion(1/2 cup cooked or 1 cup raw). It is rich in phytonutrients, which may reduce the risk of several kinds of cancer including breast, stomach, and colon.

CUCUMBER contains 1g carbs in a 50 gram portion. One-half cup of sliced cucumbers contain 2g carbs. The flesh is mostly water but also contains vitamin C and caffeic acid, both of which soothe skin irritations and reduce swelling. The skin of the cucumber is rich in fiber, magnesium, and potassium- a combination which may help lower blood pressure.

BROCCOLI RABE contains 1g carbs in a 50gram portion. One-half cup of this veggie cooked contains 3g carbs. This is an immune-boosting vegetable. A rich source of lutein and zeaxanthin, which may help prevent macular degeneration. It's also a great source of calcium, potassium, vitamin C, and bone-building vitamin K.

ICEBERG LETTUCE contains 2g of carbs in a 50gram portion. One cup of shredded iceberg lettuce contains 2g of carbs. This is an excellent source of potassium, which has been shown to lower blood pressure, and manganese which is essential for bone health and may help regulate blood sugar levels. It's also a good source of iron, calcium, magnesium, and phosphorus.

CELERY contains 2g carbs in a 50 gram portion. Two medium stalks of celery contains 2.5g of carbs. This is an excellent source of vitamin C. Also rich in nutrients which may lower cholesterol and blood pressure, and may protect against some forms of cancer by preventing damage from free radicals.

WHITE MUSHROOMS contain 2g of carbs in a 50 gram portion. One-half cup of raw slice mushrooms contain 2g of carbs. They are extremely dense with nutrients including selenium, a trace mineral that may help fight cancer. They're also rich in antioxidant and anti-inflammatory nutrients, and may help prevent cardiovascular disease.

RADISHES contain 2g of carbs in a 50 gram portion. One-half cup of sliced raw radishes contains 2g of carbs. They are an excellent source of vitamin C and calcium. They are thought to have cancer-fighting properties, and they've been used as a medicinal food for liver disorders.

TURNIPS contain 2g of carbs in a 50 gram portion. One-half cup of cooked turnips contain4g of carbs. They are especially high in cancer-fighting glucosinolates. Rich in antioxidants, including vitamin C and E, beta-carotene, and manganese. Also a good source of vitamin K and omega-3 fatty acids, both of which have anti-inflammatory properties.

ROMMAINE LETTUCE contains 2g of carbs in a 50 gram portion. One cup of shredded romaine lettuce contains 1.5g of carbs. This is an excellent source of vitamin C and beta-carotene, which works together to prevent the oxidization of cholesterol. Also rich in potassium, which lowers blood pressure. This is definitely a heart-healthy vegetable.

ASPARAGUS contains 2g of carbs in a 50 gram portion. One-half cup of cooked asparagus contains 3.5g of carbs. This is an excellent source of anti-inflammatory phytonutrients and a wide variety of antioxidant nutrients, including vitamin C, beta-carotene, zinc, manganese, and selenium. it can help reduce the risk of heart disease and regulate blood sugar because it is rich in fiber and B vitamins, which play a key role in the metabolism of sugar starches.

GREEN PEPPER contains 2g of carbs in a 50 gram portion. One-half cup of sliced green peppers contains 2g of carbs. They are a great source of vitamins C and A, and vitamin K, which is essential for bone health. Also contains folic acid which can reduce the chance of heart attack and stroke.

OKRA contains 2g of carbs in a 50 gram portion. One-half cup of cooked okra contains 3.5g of carbs. Okra is a great immune system supporter and is high in protein and fiber- one cup offers 4g fiber.

CAULIFLOWER contains 3g of carbs in a 50 gram portion. One cup of cooked cauliflower contains 5g of carbs. This is a potential cancer-fighter. It provides special nutrient support to the body's detox, antioxidant, and inflammatory system- all of which are connected to cancer development. Two cups have 6g of fiber and only 50 calories.

YELLOW PEPPER contains 3g of carbs in a 50 gram portion. One-half cup of sliced yellow pepper contains 3g of carbs. They are a good source of vitamin C and A, two powerful antioxidants, and vitamin K. Also rich in folic acid which can help prevent stroke, heart disease, dementia, and potential vascular disease.

CABBAGE contains 3g of carbs in a 50 gram portion. One cup cooked shredded cabbage contains 8.5g of carbs. Rich in antioxidants, anti-inflammatory nutrients, and glucosinolates, thought to have anti-cancer activity. Red and purple cabbage are powerful weapons against cardiovascular disease.

RED BELL PEPPER contains 3g of carbs in a 50 gram portion. One-half cup of sliced red bell pepper contains 3g of carbs. They are a good source of vitamins C and A, two powerful antioxidants, and vitamin K. Also rich in B6 and folic acid, reducing the risk of cardiovascular disease.

BROCCOLI contains 4g of carbs in a 50 gram portion. One cup of cooked broccoli contains 11g of carbs. This is a great source of isotheocyanates which are great cancer fighting agents. There are also anti-inflammatory properties in broccoli and it's a good source of fiber, which is good for digestive health.

SPINACH contains 4g of carbs in a 50 gram portion. One-half cup of cooked spinach contains 3.5g of carbs. This is one of the best sources of vitamin K, which helps build strong bones. It also contains more than a dozen flavanoid compounds that function as anti-inflammatory and cancer-fighting agents. It is a good source of antioxidants that reduce problems related to oxidative stress such as high blood pressure. Spinach also contains lutein and zeaxanthin which protect against eye disease.

BEETS contain 4g of carbs in a 50 gram portion. One-half cup of sliced canned beets contain 12.5 g of carbs. They get their color from betacyanin, which may help to prevent cancer. They also help prevent heart disease, stroke, dementia, and peripheral vascular disease.

GREEN BEANS contain 4g of carbs in a 50 gram portion. One-half cup of cooked green beans contains 5g of carbs. They are a good source of folate, a B vitamin that can help prevent heart attack, stroke, and blood clots. Green beans are also good in promoting wound healing and stimulates brain function. Helps in the metabolism of sugars, insulin, and cholesterol.

CARROTS contain 5g of carbs in a 50 gram portion. One-half cup of carrots contain 6g carbs. They are an excellent source of antioxidant compounds and the richest vegetable source of pro-vitamin A carotenes. These help protect against cardiovascular disease and cancer, and promote good vision. Carrots may be beneficial to blood sugar regulation.

KALE contains 5g of carbs in a 50 gram portion. One-half cup chopped cooked kale contains 4g of carbs. It is rich in antioxidant, anti-inflammatory, and anti-cancer nutrients. Can protect against some forms of cancer, kale is also loaded with calcium, iron, beta-carotene, vitamins A,C and K and may help prevent macular degeneration.

SUGAR SNAP PEAS contain5g of carbs in a 50 gram portion. One-half cup of whole raw sugar snap peas contains 1g of carbs. They are rich in antioxidants such as vitamin C, E, and zinc and anti-inflammatory nutrients such as omega-3 fatty acids. This combo of antioxidants and anti-inflammatory compounds may reduce the risk on inflammatory diseases, including diabetes.

ONIONS contain 7g of carbs in a 50 gram portion. One-half cup of cooked onion contains 11g of carbs. They provide many anti-inflammatory benefits and may be protective against some forms of cancer. Rich in sulfur compounds that can help lower cholesterol. They contain many triglycerides which make them a heart-healthy food.

CORN contains 10g of carbs in a 50 gram portion. One medium ear of corn contains 26g of carbs. Not really a low-carb veggie but it is rich in beta-cryptoxanthin, which lowers the risk of developing lung cancer. Contains the B vitamin pantothenic acid, which is necessary for carbohydrate, protein, and lipid metabolism.

There you go, 25 of the best vegetables for your dietary health. There is nothing at all exotic about them. You can find them easily in any grocery store or produce market. You may even want to try your hand at gardening and raising your own fresh produce! Enjoy these vegetables and appreciate all the benefits nature's bounty has to offer.

Chapter 5

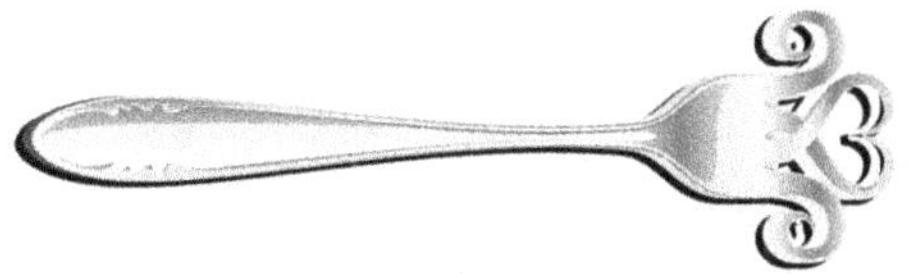

~DIABETICS HEALTHY TIPS~

As I close out the information section of this book, I'd like to offer some very healthy tips to help you on your journey. Choosing to live a healthy lifestyle can be confusing in the beginning, but if you keep a few things in mind, it can become a part of who you are and what you want to become. Always stay focused on what you want to feel like and how you want to look. If you can vision yourself vibrant and healthy, then you can become just that!

We are not all equal when it comes to health, but we can all take care of ourselves and dedicate our lives to being the very best person possible. No matter what you feel like right now, no matter how you look- you must remember that you are worthy of living a happy and healthy life. You deserve every good thing that God has for you. Don't allow illness or appearance to take control over you. Take charge of your life one step at a time, one meal at a time, and one day at a time. Did you know it takes 30 days to create a habit? If you can do just one healthy thing for 30 days, it will become a habit for you! Once you create one healthy change, add another. Before you know it, you will be living a much healthier life, taking walks, dancing, and eating better foods. Never look at it as a "job" or a "diet". Those words alone sound horrible. Look at it as a new lifestyle, a better way of living. Create the healthy life that you were meant to have. You can do it, I believe in you!

With that being said, let's move on to the healthy tips that I really want you to remember.

Tip #1: Choose high-fiber, slow-release carbohydrates.

Carbs have a big impact on your blood sugar levels- more than fats and proteins- but you don't have to avoid them. You just need to be smart about what type of carbs you eat. It's best to limit highly refined carbohydrates like white bread, pasta, and rice, as well as soda, candy, and snack foods. Instead, focus on high-fiber complex carbohydrates, also known as slow-release carbs. They help keep blood sugar levels even because they are digested more slowly, thus preventing your body from producing too much insulin. They also provide lasting energy and help you stay full longer. Here is a list of substitutions you may want to try:

Instead of...	Try this...
White rice	Brown or wild rice
White potatoes	Sweet potatoes/winter squash
Regular pasta	Whole-wheat pasta
White bread	Whole wheat/whole grain bread
Sugary breakfast cereal	High-fiber cereal (Raisin Bran)
Instant Oatmeal	Steel cut/rolled oats
Croissant/Pastry	Bran Muffin

The 8 Principles of Low Glycemc Eating

1. Eat lots of non-starchy vegetables, beans, and fruits such as apples, pears, peaches, and berries. Even tropical fruits like bananas, mangoes, and papayas tend to have a lower glycemic index than typical desserts.

2. Eat grains in the least-processed state as possible, such as whole kernel bread, brown rice, and whole barley, millet, and wheat berries, steel cut oats, and natural granola or muesli breakfast cereals.
3. Limit white potatoes and refined grain products such as white breads and white pasta to small side dishes.
4. Limit concentrated sweets including high-calorie foods with a low glycemic index, such as ice cream, to occasional treats. Reduce fruit juice to no more than one cup a day. Completely eliminate sugar-sweetened drinks.
5. Eat a healthy protein at most meals, such as beans, fish, or skinless chicken.
6. Choose foods with healthy fats, such as olive oil, nuts (almonds, walnuts, pecans), and avocados. Limit saturated fats from dairy and other animal products. Completely eliminate trans fats (partially hydrogenated fats), which are found in fast foods and many processed foods.
7. Have three meals and one or two snacks every day. Never skip breakfast!
8. Eat slowly, and stop when you are full. You don't need to "stuff" yourself. When you begin to feel full, that's the stopping point.

Tip #2: Think smart about sweets.

Just because you are Diabetic does not mean you have to eliminate sugar completely. You can still enjoy a small serving of your favorite dessert once in awhile. The key is "moderation"! Maybe you have a sweet tooth and the thought of cutting back on sweets sounds almost as bad as cutting them out altogether. The good news is that cravings do go away, and your food preferences will actually change over time. As your eating habits become healthier, you'll find that foods you used to love may seem too rich or too sweet for you now, and you will find yourself craving the healthier options now.

The big question I get more often is, how to include sweets in a Diabetic-friendly diet? Here are some useful points to remember:

- **Skip the bread, rice, or pasta if you want dessert.** Eating sweets at a meal adds extra carbohydrates. Because of this, it is best to cut back on the other carbs in that same meal.

- **Add some healthy fat to your dessert.** It may seem crazy to pass over the low-fat or fat-free desserts and choose the higher-fat option. But actually fat slows down the digestive process, meaning blood sugar levels don't spike as quickly! Now that doesn't mean that you should eat a glazed donut. Think HEALTHY fats, such as peanut butter, ricotta cheese, yogurt, or some nuts. A good yogurt and fruit parfait makes a great dessert. Even a peanut butter cookie is sufficient here. Just remember...keep sugars under control.

- **Eat sweets with a meal rather than a stand-alone snack.** When eaten alone, sweets tend to make your blood sugars spike. But if you eat them along with other healthy foods as part of your meal, your blood sugar won't spike as rapidly.

- **When you eat dessert, truly savor each bite.** Sometimes it's easy to mindlessly eat your way through a bag of cookies or a huge piece of cake. Can you say that you really savored each bite? Make your indulgence count by eating and paying attention to the flavors and textures of your dessert. You'll enjoy it more, and you're less likely to overeat. Don't scoff down a bag of cookies, you know better than that. Just enjoy a small portion of your dessert by slowing down and basking in the flavor!

How do you cut down on sugar?

- **Reduce your soda and juice intake.** If you miss the bubbles from carbonated drinks, try sparkling water either plain or with a little juice mixed in!
- **Reduce the amount of sugars in recipes** by 1/4 to 1/3. If a recipe calls for 1 cup of sugar, use 2/3 or 3/4 cup instead. You can also boost sweetness with cinnamon, nutmeg, or vanilla extract.
- **Find healthy ways to satisfy your sweet tooth.** Instead of ice cream, blend up some frozen banana slices for a creamy frozen treat that tastes amazingly like ice cream! (Peel them before freezing or you'll never get the skin off!). Enjoy a small chunk of dark chocolate instead of your favorite milk chocolate bar.
- **Start with half of the dessert you normally eat,** and replace the other half with fresh fruit.

Watch the alcohol

Many people often underestimate the number of calories in alcoholic drinks, including beer and wine. Cocktails mixed with soda and juice can be loaded with sugar. If you are going to drink, please do so in moderation (no more than 1 drink per day for women; two for men), choose calorie-free drink mixers, and drink only with food. If you're Diabetic, always remember to monitor your blood glucose, as alcohol can really interfere with your medications and insulin. I say don't drink at all, but if you must do it, please take these precautions.

Tip #3: Choose fats wisely.

Fats can be helpful or harmful to your diet. Diabetics are at higher risk for heart disease, so it's even more important to be smart about fats. As I stated earlier, some fats are unhealthy and some have enormous health benefits. But remember, all fats are high in calories, so you still need to watch your portion sizes.

How to reduce unhealthy fats and add healthy fats:

Cook with olive oil instead of butter or vegetable oil.

- Trim any visible fat off of meat before cooking and remove the skin off chicken or turkey before cooking.
- Replace chips and crackers with nuts or seeds. Add them to your morning cereal or enjoy a handful for a snack.
- Instead of frying, choose to grill, bake, broil, or stir-fry.
- Replace red meat with fish 2-3 time per week.
- Add avocado to your sandwich in place of cheese. You'll still have the creamy texture while adding health benefits.
- Use canola oil or applesauce when baking, in place of shortening or butter.
- Replace heavy cream in soups by adding pureed tomatoes or reduced fat sour cream!

Tip #4: Eat regularly and keep a food diary

If you are overweight, I have some encouraging news for you. You only have to lose 7% of your body weight to cut your risk of Diabetes in half! And you don't have to tirelessly count calories or starve yourself to do it. When it comes to successful weight loss, the two most helpful strategies involve following a regular eating schedule and recording what you eat. Your body is better able to regulate blood sugar levels- and your weight- when you maintain a regular meal schedule. Your goal is to maintain moderate and consistent portion sizes for each meal or snack.

- Do not skip breakfast. Eating a good breakfast daily will give you the energy you need to jumpstart your day as well as help keep blood sugar levels steady.
- Eat regular small meals - up to 6 per day. We tend to eat more when we are really hungry. Eating regularly will keep your portions in check.
- Keep calorie intake the same. Try to eat roughly the same amount of calories each day at each meal, rather than over eating during one meal and barely eating for another. Consistency is key.
- Keep a food diary. When you actually look at what you are putting in your body, it's easier to pin-point where your problem areas or weaknesses may be. You may find that you can cut back in some areas by using the substitution method - replacing some foods with healthier choices.

Don't forget the exercise!

This is the part that no one wants to talk about. But no matter how you look at it, exercise is vital when it comes to being healthy. When it comes to preventing, controlling, or reversing Diabetes, you can't overlook exercise! It can help your weight loss efforts, and is especially important in maintaining weight loss. Regular exercise can even improve your insulin sensitivity even if you don't lose weight!

I'm not saying you have to get a gym membership right away or adopt a grueling fitness regimen in the next day or two, but you do need to get your body in motion in some way. A good start for anyone on any level is to:

- Start the morning with a good stretch. This wakes up your whole body and gets the blood flowing. Stretch the legs, arms, and waist.
- Walk for 30 minutes at least 5 times a week. Take a stroll through the neighborhood or at your local park. I always like listening to my favorite music while I walk, it makes the time go by and I really enjoy it!
- Try biking or swimming.
- Do a little weight-training. Get a set of dumb bells to strengthen your arms. Or you can use detergent bottles filled with sand, water, or rocks!
- Try a few push-ups and sit ups. Do what your body can handle, and slowly increase them.
- Yard work! You can get lots of real good exercise by working right in the yard. Raking leaves, pushing a mower, pruning plants, etc. will give you a good work-out. Plant a garden or some flowers. This will give you a reason to consistently work outside. Plus the beautiful benefits will make you feel good. Enjoy the flowers and/or the fresh veggies.

Remember that the whole point in exercising is to burn calories and tone up. You want to break a sweat each time, so get a towel and let the perspiration be your guide.

Success signs for a good workout: increased heart rate, harder breathing, and sweat! Don't look at it as a "task". Picture a healthier you. Think of how many years you are adding to your life, the quality of living, and the end results. You deserve to feel good, look good, and live a fulfilling life! I truly believe that you are capable of doing this.

Now that we've covered all the technical stuff, it's time to get to the good part. My favorite part, of course, is sharing the recipes. I have worked, researched, tested, and tasted so many recipes for healthier living. Some were good, some were terrible, and some were definitely keepers. I wanted to offer recipes that Diabetics could enjoy, but I also wanted them to be tasty enough for the entire family. This next section is filled with recipes that can be appreciated by anyone who wants to eat healthy.

You definitely don't have to be Diabetic to enjoy these healthy, tasty dishes. I'm sure that you and your loved ones will have fun creating these fabulous meals. Believe me, being Diabetic doesn't mean you have to sacrifice flavor in your favorite foods.

I also have a few Vegetarian and Gluten-Free recipes for some of my other friends with special dietary requests.

Let's get to it!

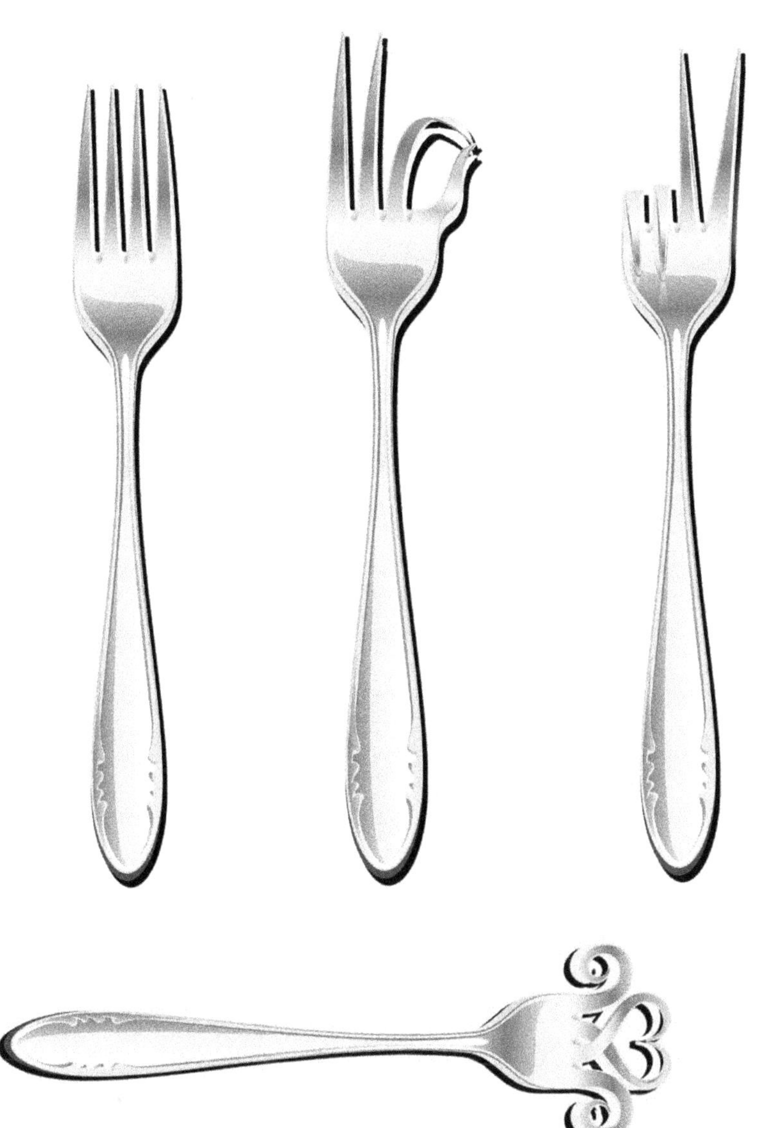

Chapter 6

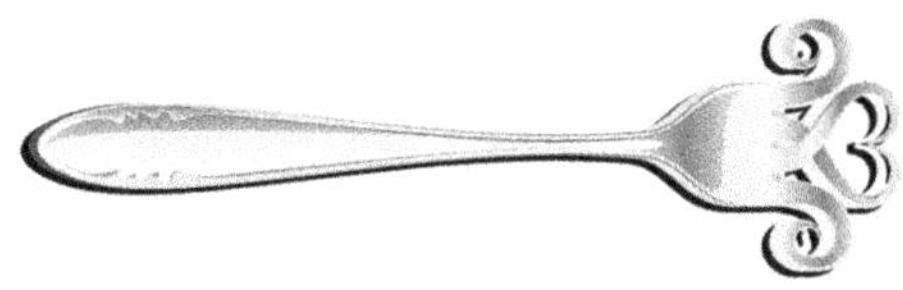

~DIABETIC APPETIZERS~

SIMPLE GUACAMOLE

1 medium avocado
1 Tbsp. salsa
1 medium clove of garlic, peeled
1/4 tsp. salt
1/4 tsp white pepper
1 tsp. fresh lime juice

Process all ingredients in a blender or food processor. Leave it a little chunky for texture. Spoon into your serving bowl and serve. Makes 6 servings, 2 Tbsp. each.

Calories: 45, Total Carbs: 2.8g, Dietary Fiber: 0.8g, Sugars: 0.1g, Total Fat: 3.8g, Saturated Fat: 0.4g, Unsaturated Fat: 3.4g, Potassium: 121.3mg, Protein 0.8g, Sodium 111.5 mg, Dietary Exchanges: 1 Fat

DELICIOUS HONEY-ALMOND SPREAD

1/4 cup raw almonds, finely ground
2 oz. honey
4 tsp. cold water
1 pinch salt

Blend all the ingredients in a blender until smooth and spreadable. Serve on your favorite wheat crackers or even with raw fruit or veggies. Makes 8 servings.

Calories: 20.6, Total Carbs: 1.5g, Dietary Fiber: 0.4g, Sugars: 0.9g, Total Fat: 1.5g, Saturated Fat 0.1 g, Unsaturated Fat: 1.4g, Potassium: 21.2 mg, Protein: 0.6g, Sodium: 0.2 mg, Dietary Exchanges: 1/4 Fat

ORANGES WITH DATES

3 medium navel oranges
2 dates, cut into strips
1 Tbsp. honey

Peel the oranges and cut them crosswise into 1/4 inch slices. Put them on your serving plate and toss the sliced dates over the top. Drizzle with honey. Makes 4 servings.

Calories: 63.4, Total Carbs: 18.7g, Dietary Fiber: 5.5g, Sugars: 13.1g, Total Fat: 0g, Saturated Fat: 0g, Unsaturated Fat: 0g, Potassium: 187.5mg, Protein: 0.8g, Sodium: 0mg, Dietary Exchanges: 1 fruit

TASTY TOMATO BRUSCHETTA

2 oz. anchovy fillets, rinse and drain
2 tsp. capers, drained
3 fresh plum tomatoes, seeded and chopped
1 Tbsp. onion, chopped
1 Tbsp. fresh parsley, chopped
1/4 cup fresh Romano cheese, grated
6 slices Italian bread, sliced

Preheat your oven to 350 degrees. Pat the rinsed and drained anchovies dry with some paper towel. Chop the anchovies and put them in a small bowl along with the capers, tomatoes, onion, parsley, and grated cheese. Place the bread on a baking sheet and lightly toast both sides. Spread your topping over the toasted bread and serve. Makes about 6 servings.

Calories: 82.1, Total Carbs: 11.5g, Dietary Fiber: 1g, Sugars: 1.1g, Total Fat: 2.1g, Saturated Fat: 1.1g, Unsaturated Fat: 1g, Potassium: 110.9mg, Protein: 3.8g, Sodium: 291.2mg, Dietary Exchanges: 1 Starch, 1/4 Vegetable, 1/4 Very Lean Meat

HEAVENLY DEVILLED EGGS

6 large eggs
1/4 cup cottage cheese
3 Tbsp. ranch dressing
2 tsp. Dijon mustard
2 Tbsp. minced chives
1 Tbsp. pimento, drained and diced
4 cups cold water, divided

Place eggs in a medium size saucepan. Add enough water to completely cover the eggs. Bring to a rolling boil over medium heat. Cover and turn off the heat and allow to sit 15 minutes. Drain off the hot water and add cold water to cool the eggs. Drain and peel eggs. Cut the eggs in half, lengthwise, and remove the yolks. Reserve 3 yolks and save the others for another use. Place the egg whites on serving plate and cover with some plastic wrap while you make the filling. Combine the 3 yolks with cottage cheese and ranch dressing, stir until smooth. Add the chives and pimento. Mix well and spoon into the egg whites. Cover and chill at least one hour. Makes 4 servings.

Calories: 179.6, Total Carbs: 1.8g, Dietary Fiber: 0.1g, Sugars: 1.2g, Total Fat: 14.4g, Saturated Fat 3.6g, Unsaturated Fat: 10.8g, Potassium: 109.7mg, Protein: 11.1g, Sodium 303.7mg, Dietary Exchanges: 1 1/2 Fat, 1/2 Meat

Sharon Fox

EASY CREAMY ARTICHOKE DIP

1/2 cup fat-free sour cream
1/2 cup light mayonnaise
1 envelope Light Italian Salad Dressing Mix
14 oz. canned artichoke hearts, drained and chopped finely

In a medium size bowl mix the sour cream, mayonnaise, Italian dressing mix, and artichoke hearts together. Refrigerate until ready to serve.
Makes 12 servings, 1 Tbsp. each.

Calories: 58.5, Total Carbs: 5.9g, Dietary Fiber: 2.4g, Sugars: 1.4g, Total Fat: 3.3g, Saturated Fat: 0.5g, Unsaturated Fat: 2.8g, Potassium: 103.5mg, Protein: 1.5g, Sodium: 133.7mg, Dietary Exchanges: 1 Fat, 1/2 Vegetable

ASPARAGUS SQUARES

1 cup chopped Vidalia onion
2 medium cloves garlic, minced
3 Tbsp. unsalted butter
1 lb. fresh asparagus, ends trimmed off
1/4 tsp. black pepper
2 - 8oz. tubes refrigerated Crescent roll dough
1 cup part skim mozzarella shredded cheese
1 cup shredded Swiss cheese

In a large skillet, saute the onion in butter until tender. Add the garlic and cook one minute longer, being very careful not to burn. Cut the asparagus into 1 inch pieces, set the tips aside. Add the remaining asparagus to the skillet and saute until crisp-tender. Add the asparagus tips and pepper. Stir and cook 1-2 minutes until asparagus is tender.
Press the Crescent roll dough into an ungreased 15x10x1-inch baking pan, sealing the perforations and seams. Bake at 375 degrees until lightly browned, about 7 minutes. Top with the asparagus mixture and then sprinkle with cheeses. Bake 7 minutes longer or until the cheese is melted. Cut into squares. Makes 3 dozen. Serving size is one square.

Calories: 84, Total Carbs: 6.3g, Dietary Fiber: 0.4g, Sugars: 1.4g, Total Fat: 5.0g, Saturated Fat: 2.1g, Unsaturated Fat: 2.9g, Potassium: 40mg, Protein: 2.9g, Sodium: 125.6mg, Dietary Exchanges: 1/4 Fat, 1/4 Starch

AVOCADO AND PEAR DIP

2 avocadoes, peeled, pitted, and mashed
1 large pear, peeled and diced
2 green onions finely chopped, white and green parts
1 jalapeno, minced (remove seeds if you don't want it too hot)
3 Tbsp. fresh lime juice
1 pinch salt

In blender, combine all ingredients and blend until smooth. Scrape the sides at least once to combine well. Transfer to serving bowl and cover with plastic wrap. Refrigerate for a half hour before serving. Serve with low-carb, whole grain chips or vegetable sticks. Makes 10 servings, 3oz. each.

Be sure to wear gloves when working with jalapeno peppers. Avoid touching your eyes!

Calories: 80.2, Total Carbs: 7.7g, Dietary Fiber: 3.5g, Sugars 2.7g, Total Fat: 5.9g, Saturated Fat: 0.8g, Unsaturated Fat: 5.1g, Potassium: 239.3mg, Protein: 1g, Sodium: 14.2mg, Dietary Exchanges: 1 1/4 Fat

PINEAPPLE AND AVOCADO SALSA

1 fresh pineapple, peeled and diced
1 medium avocado, peeled and diced
1/3 cup red onion, chopped
4 stalks celery, finely chopped
1 jalapeno, seeded and chopped
3 Tbsp. fresh lime juice
1 tsp. lime zest
1/4 tsp. salt

Combine all ingredients in a bowl. Cover with plastic wrap and chill at least 30 minutes before serving. Serve with baked chips. Makes 20 servings.

Calories: 28.7, Total Carbs: 5g, Dietary Fiber: 0.9g, Sugars: 2.5g, Total Fat: 1.1g, Saturated Fat: 0.1g, Unsaturated Fat: 1g, Potassium: 70.3mg, Protein: 0.6g, Sodium: 42mg, Dietary Exchanges: 1/4 Fat

CHEDDAR-BACON STUFFED MUSHROOMS

3 slices bacon, cooked, drained, and crumbled
3/4 cup Crimini mushrooms
1 Tbsp. butter
1 Tbsp. chopped red onion
3/4 cup shredded cheddar cheese

Preheat the oven to 400 degrees. Fry bacon, drain and set aside. Remove the mushroom stems, set aside the caps. Finely chop the stems. In a large saucepan over medium heat, melt the butter. Slowly cook the diced stems and onion, stirring occasionally until the onion is soft.
In a medium bowl, stir together the mushroom stem/onion mixture, crumbled bacon, and 1/2 cup of the shredded cheese. Scoop the mixture into the mushroom caps. Top with the remaining shredded cheddar cheese. Bake for 15 minutes, or until the cheese has melted. Makes 8 servings.

Calories: 94, Total Carbs: 0.6g, Dietary Fiber: 0g, Sugars: 0.1g, Total Fat: 8.6g, Saturated Fat: 4g, Unsaturated Fat: 4.6g, Potassium: 55.6mg, Protein: 3.7g, Sodium: 148.6mg, Dietary Exchanges: 1 1/4 Fat, 1/2 Meat

BLT PARTY BRUSCHETTA

8 slices bacon, cooked crispy and crumbled
1 1/3 cups Roma tomatoes, seeded and chopped
1 cup shredded lettuce
2 Tbsp. fresh basil, chopped
1 garlic clove, minced
1/4 tsp. salt
1/4 tsp. black pepper
1/3 cup olive oil, to brush over bread slices
French baguette bread, sliced into 24 slices
1/3 cup crumbled blue cheese (feta or goat cheese may be used)

In a medium bowl, combine all the topping ingredients and set aside. Brush olive oil over each slice of bread on both sides and place on a baking sheet. Bake in a 400 degree oven for 7 minutes on each side, or until golden brown, and allow to cool. Spoon about 1 Tbsp. of the topping onto each toast. Makes 24 servings.

Calories: 67.5, Total Carbs: 5.2g, Dietary Fiber: 0.4g, Sugars: 0.5g, Total Fat: 4.3g, Saturated Fat: 0.8g, Unsaturated Fat: 3.5g, Potassium 40.4mg, Protein: 1.9g, Sodium: 148.4mg, Dietary Exchanges: 1 Fat, 1/4 Starch

PIGGY-BACK DATES

12 slices of low-sodium bacon
24 pitted dates

Cut bacon slices in half and fully wrap each pitted date with each half. Secure the bacon using toothpicks that have been soaked in water for 15 minutes. Soaking the toothpicks will keep them from burning. Bake on a parchment lined baking sheet for about 10-15 minutes, or until the bacon has cooked completely. Cool for 10 minutes before serving. Makes 24 servings.

Calories: 67.5, Total Carbs: 5.2g, Dietary Fiber: 0.4g, Sugars: 0.5g, Total Fat: 4.3g, Saturated Fat: 0.8g, Unsaturated Fat: 3.5g, Potassium: 40.4mg, Protein: 1.9g, Sodium: 148.4mg, Dietary Exchanges: 1 Fat, 1/4 Starch

OLIVE CREAM CHEESE SPREAD

8 oz. fat-free cream cheese, softened
4 Tbsp. low-fat sour cream
2-3 cloves garlic cloves, minced
3 oz. stuffed green olives, chopped (reserve 1 tsp. liquid from the jar)
1 tsp. Italian seasoning
1 tsp. fresh chives, finely chopped

Combine all ingredients, stirring in the 1 tsp. of the liquid from the jar of olives. Chill until ready to serve. Spread on bagel chips or whole wheat crackers. Makes 8 servings.

Nutrition info does not include the bagel chips or crackers.

Calories: 72.5, Total Carbs: 9g, Dietary Fiber: 0.3g, Sugars: 0.8g, Total Fat: 1.7g, Saturated Fat: 0.3g, Unsaturated Fat: 1.4g, Potassium: 58.6mg, Protein: 5.4g, Sodium: 403.9mg, Dietary Exchanges: 1/2 starch.

BAKED CRAB DIP

1 cup green onion, chopped
2 Tbsp. chopped parsley
2 Tbsp. chopped celery
3 Tbsp. unsalted margarine, 80% fat
3 Tbsp. all-purpose flour
pinch of salt and pepper
1 1/2 cup fat-free milk
1 Tbsp. cooking sherry
1 1.2 lb raw Blue crab
1 cup reduced-fat cheddar cheese, finely shredded

Preheat oven to 375 degrees. In a saucepan, melt margarine and saute the green onions, celery, and parsley until tender. Stir in the flour, salt, and pepper. Gradually stir in milk, stirring over low heat until the mixture is thick and bubbly. Remove from heat and add the cooking sherry. Gently fold in the crab meat. Place into a casserole dish or divide into 6 individual serving size ramekins. Sprinkle cheese over the top and bake 10-15 minutes until cheese is melted and slightly browned. Makes 6 servings.

Calories: 257, Total Carbs: 7.8g, Dietary Fiber: 0.2g, Sugars: 3.7g, Total Fat: 11.1g, Saturated Fat: 3.7g, Unsaturated Fat: 7.4g, Potassium: 91.4mg, Protein: 30.7g, Sodium: 567mg, Dietary Exchanges: 1 1/4 Fat, 1 Meat, 1/4 Milk, 3 1/4 Very Lean Meat.

BAKED GREEN TOMATOES

1 cup cornmeal or whole-wheat dry bread crumbs
1 Tbsp. dried dill weed
1 tsp. garlic powder
1 pinch salt
1 pinch black pepper
1/2 cup egg whites
5 green tomatoes, thinly sliced
olive oil cooking spray

Preheat your oven to 350 degrees. Lightly grease a baking sheet.

In a small bowl, combine the cornmeal (or bread crumbs), dill, garlic powder, salt, and pepper. Dip each tomato slice into egg whites and then crumb mixture, coating both sides. Arrange in a single layer on prepared baking sheet. Spray tomatoes with olive oil spray and bake 15 minutes. Turn them over, spray this side with olive oil spray as well and bake for another 15-20 minutes, until golden brown. Spraying them with olive oil spray with make them crispy! Makes 6 servings.

Calories: 80.1, Total Carbs: 16.9g, Dietary Fiber: 3.6g, Sugars: 4.1g, Total Fat: 0.6g, Saturated Fat: 0g, Unsaturated Fat: 0.6g, Potassium: 276.1mg, Protein: 2.9g, Sodium: 36.1mg, Dietary Exchanges: 1 Vegetable.

BAKED POTATO DIP

2- 16 oz. containers sour cream
3 oz. vegetarian meat bacon bits
2 cups sharp cheddar cheese, shredded
1 bunch green onions, chopped (green and white parts)

In a medium size mixing bowl, combine the sour cream, vegetarian bacon bits, shredded cheese, and green onions. Mix well. Cover and refrigerate for 1 hour before serving.

Great served on a vegetable tray with carrot and celery sticks, and red and yellow bell pepper strips! Makes 32 servings.

Calories: 85.1, Total Carbs: 2.2g, Dietary Fiber: 0g, Sugars: 1g, Total Fat: 7g, Saturated Fat: 4.6g, Unsaturated Fat: 2.4g, Potassium: 6.5mg, Protein: 2.8g, Sodium: 90.4mg, Dietary Exchanges: 1 Fat, 1/4 Meat.

Nutrition Information is only for the dip.

BAKED SHRIMP FOR TWO

1/2 lb. raw medium shrimp, shelled and deveined
1 Tbsp. unsalted butter
1 clove garlic, minced
1 tsp. fresh lemon juice
1 Tbsp. chopped parsley
1 tsp. grated Parmesan cheese

Preheat the oven to 350 degrees. In a small saucepan, place the butter, garlic, lemon juice, and parsley. Simmer over low heat to melt the butter and soften the garlic. Rinse shrimp and put them in a small casserole dish. Pour the melted butter mixture over the shrimp. Cover and bake 10-12 minutes. Remove from oven and sprinkle with Parmesan cheese. Makes 2 4 oz. servings.

Calories: 200.3, Total Carbs: 2g, Dietary Fiber: 0.1g, Sugars: 0.1g, Total Fat: 8.5g, Saturated Fat: 4.2g, Unsaturated Fat: 4.3g, Potassium: 28mg, Protein: 26.7g, Sodium: 213.4mg, Dietary Exchanges: 1 1/4 Fat, 4 Very Lean Meat.

BAKED OYSTERS ON THE HALF SHELL

1 1/2 slices soft white bread
cooking spray
1/3 cup green onions, chopped
2 cloves garlic, minced
1/3 cup seasoned Italian dry bread crumbs
1/4 cup grated Parmesan cheese
1 tsp. fresh lemon juice
1/8 tsp. ground cayenne (red pepper)
1/8 tsp. black pepper
12 medium oysters, shucked (24 on the half shell)
4 lemons

Preheat oven to 450 degrees. Use a food processor to blend white bread to create rough bread crumbs- should measure out to 3/4 cup. Heat a medium skillet, coated with cooking spray, over medium heat. To the skillet, add onions, parsley, and garlic. Stir and cook for about 5 minutes. Remove from heat and add the white bread crumbs, Italian bread crumbs, cheese, lemon juice, cayenne, and black pepper. Arrange oysters on a baking sheet and divide mixture equally onto each oyster. Place in the oven and bake about 6-7 minutes, the edges of the oysters should curl. Garnish with lemon wedges. This recipe also works with clams. Makes 8 servings.

Calories: 129.1, Total Carbs: 14.1g, Dietary Fiber: 0.7g, Sugars: 1.5g, Total Fat: 3.6g, Saturated Fat: 1.3g, Unsaturated Fat: 2.3g, Potassium: 146.8mg, Protein: 9.7g, Sodium: 376.5mg, Dietary Exchanges: 1 1/4 Meat, 1/2 Starch.

SPINACH BALLS WITH HONEY MUSTARD SAUCE

2 cups Pepperidge Farm dry Herb Stuffing
1/4 cup reduced fat grated Parmesan cheese
1/4 cup green onion, chopped
2 garlic cloves, minced
1/8 tsp. ground nutmeg
10 oz. frozen spinach, thawed and drained
1/4 cup low-sodium vegetable broth
2 Tbsp. butter, melted
a pinch of salt and pepper
2 egg whites, lightly beaten

Sauce:
3/4 cup fat-free sour cream
1 Tbsp. Dijon mustard
1 Tbsp. fresh chives, chopped
1 1/2 Tbsp. honey

In a medium size bowl, combine the dry stuffing, Parmesan cheese, onions, garlic, and nutmeg. Mix in the spinach, vegetable broth, and butter. Season with salt and pepper. Stir in the egg whites and mix well.

Shape the mixture into 24 balls. Place on a greased baking sheet and bake at 350 degrees until browned, about 15 minutes. While they're baking, make the sauce by combining all the sauce ingredients in a bowl. Makes 12 servings.

Calories: 88.3, Total Carbs: 12.2g, Dietary Fiber: 0.9g, Sugars: 3.7g, Total Fat: 2.6g, Saturated Fat: 0.6g, Unsaturated Fat: 2g, Potassium: 13.2mg, Protein: 3.5g, Sodium: 273.5mg, Dietary Exchanges: 1/2 Fat, 1/2 Starch.

EASY BAKED CRAB CAKES

1 1/2 lbs. raw Blue crab, cartilage and shells removed
2 Tbsp. mayonnaise
2 Tbsp. Dijon mustard
3 Tbsp. yellow onion, minced
1 egg
cooking spray

Preheat broiler. Lightly coat baking pan with cooking spray. Combine all ingredients in a medium mixing bowl. Mix lightly, trying not to break up all the crab meat. Shape into 6 equal patties and place on the prepared baking pan. Place under broiler at least 6 inches from the heat. Cook for 3 minutes on each side, until lightly browned. Makes 6 servings.

Calories: 165.7, Total Carbs: 1.8g, Dietary Fiber: 0.1g, Sugars: 0.4g, Total Fat: 5.9g, Saturated Fat: 1g., Unsaturated Fat: 4.9g, Potassium: 100.9mg, Protein: 24.4g, Sodium: 534mg, Dietary Exchanges: 1 Fat, 3 1/4 Very Lean Meat.

LOUISIANA SHRIMP KABOBS

1 1/2 Tbsp. ground paprika
1/8 tsp. ground thyme
1 tsp. oregano
1 1/2 tsp. garlic powder
1 1/2 tsp. brown sugar
1 tsp. onion powder
1 tsp. black pepper
1/2 tsp. salt
1/4 tsp. cayenne (ground red pepper)
1 lb. large raw shrimp, shelled and deveined (about 40)
1 Tbsp. extra virgin olive oil
cooking spray
1/4 cup celery salt

Soak 10 wooden skewers in water for 30 minutes before grilling to prevent burning. Preheat grill to medium-high or preheat broiler. In a small bowl, combine the paprika, thyme, oregano, garlic powder, brown sugar, onion powder, black pepper, salt, cayenne pepper, and celery salt. In a large bowl, place the shrimp and sprinkle with the spice mixture. Toss with your hands to coat each shrimp. Drizzle with olive oil and toss again. Thread 4 shrimp on each skewer by bending each one so the ends are nearly touching and skewer goes through each shrimp twice. Coat grill or broiler pan with cooking spray. Grill or broil for 3 minutes on each side, until shrimp are caramelized and done. Makes 10 servings.

Calories: 35.3, Total Carbs: 2g, Dietary Fiber: 0.6g, Sugars: 0.6g, Total Fat 1.7g, Saturated Fat: 0.2g, Unsaturated Fat: 1.5g, Potassium: 97.9mg, Protein: 2.9g, Sodium: 602.2mg, Dietary Exchanges: 1/4 Fat, 1/4 Very Lean Meat

CANTALOUPE SOUP

2 cantaloupe (3 lbs. each), chopped
1 individual size plain or vanilla yogurt (Yoplait is my choice)
3 Tbsp. fresh lemon juice
1 tsp. balsamic vinegar
2 Tbsp. honey
1/2 tsp. fresh rosemary, chopped
1/2 tsp. cinnamon
1/4 tsp. black pepper
1/4 tsp. salt

Blend the cantaloupe in a blender until smooth. Add the remaining ingredients and process until smooth. Refrigerate until ready to serve. Makes 8 servings.

Calories: 66.7, Total Carbs: 14.9g, Dietary Fiber: 1.1g, Sugars: 13.2g, Total Fat: 0g, Saturated Fats 0g, Unsaturated Fat 0g, Potassium 8.8mg, Protein 2.4g, Sodium: 119.2mg, Dietary Exchanges: 1 fruit.

LIGHT CHEESE FONDUE

1 1/2 cups dry white wine
3 large cloves of garlic, peeled
8 oz. fat-free cream cheese
2 cups low-fat Swiss cheese, shredded
1 Tbsp. all purpose flour
1 pinch each of salt, pepper, and cayenne (red pepper)

Combine the wine and garlic in a pot and bring to a boil. Lower the heat and simmer until it reduces to 3/4 cup. Discard the garlic. Stir in the cream cheese and cook until it melts completely. Combine the Swiss cheese and flour in a bowl. Stir the cheese/flour into the sauce and stir continually until melted. Sprinkle with the salt, pepper, and cayenne. Serve in a fondue pot with bread cubes or vegetables for dipping. Makes 8 servings, 1/4 cup each.

Calories: 107.3, Total Carbs: 4.1g, Dietary Fiber: 0g, Sugars: 0.8g, Total Fat: 1.9g, Saturated Fat 1g, Unsaturated Fat: 0.9g, Potassium: 82.3mg, Protein: 9g, Sodium: 130.4mg, Dietary Exchanges: 1/2 Fat, 1 Meat

CRISPY CHEESY WONTON CHIPS

10 wonton wrappers
2 Tbsp. grated Parmesan cheese
2 tsp. olive oil
1/8 tsp. garlic powder

Spray a baking sheet with cooking spray and preheat oven to 375 degrees. Cut each wonton wrapper diagonally in half to form 2 triangles. Place them in a single layer on the baking sheet.

In a small bowl, combine the cheese with oil and garlic powder. Sprinkle over the wonton triangles. Bake for 6-8 minutes, until golden brown and crispy. Remove from oven and cool completely. Makes 4 servings. This will satisfy that craving for potato chips!

Calories: 75.2, Total Carbs: 7.8g, Dietary Fiber: 0.3g, Sugars: 0.2g, Total Fat: 3.5g, Saturated Fat: 1.1g, Unsaturated Fat: 2.4g, Potassium 0mg, Protein: 3g, Sodium: 156.4mg, Dietary Exchanges: 1/2 Fat, 1/2 Starch.

CHICKEN-N-BACON BITES

2 boneless skinless chicken breasts, cut into 32 bite size pieces
1/3 cup fat-free white wine vinaigrette salad dressing
16 slices bacon, cut in half crosswise
32 toothpicks, soaked 30 minutes in water

Preheat oven to 425 degrees. Marinate the chicken in the vinaigrette for 30 minutes. Wrap each chicken piece with bacon, secure with a toothpick. Place on a foil lined cookie sheet and bake 15- 20 minutes until cooked through. Makes 32 servings.

Calories: 63, Total Carbs: 0.9, Dietary Fiber: 0g, Sugars: 0.5g, Total Fat: 5.2g, Saturated Fat: 1.7g, Unsaturated Fat: 3.5g, Potassium: 42.4mg, Protein: 3g, Sodium: 124.5mg, Dietary Exchanges 1 Fat.

NOTES

Chapter 7

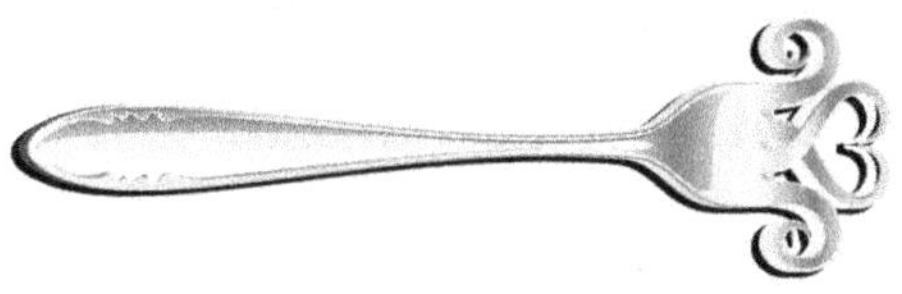

~DIABETIC BREAKFAST& Brunch~

BLUEBERRY AND ALMOND PANCAKES

1/2 cup white whole wheat flour
3/4 cup whole wheat flour
2 tsp. frozen apple juice concentrate, thawed
2 tsp. baking powder
1/4 tsp. salt
1 1/2 tsp. unsweetened applesauce
1 1/4 cup whole milk
1/8 tsp. almond extract
3 egg whites
3/4 cup fresh blueberries (frozen may be used)
1 Tbsp. slivered almonds, crushed
cooking spray

In a large bowl, combine the flours, apple juice concentrate, baking powder, and salt. In another bowl, combine the applesauce, milk, almond extract, egg whites, blueberries, and almonds. Add the flour mixture to the liquid mixture and combine until smooth. Spray your griddle or skillet with cooking spray. Heat to medium and pour 1/4 cup of the batter for each pancake. Cook each side until golden brown. Makes 8 servings.

Calories: 113, Total Carbs: 18.9g, Dietary Fiber: 2.7g, Sugars 4.4g, Total Fat: 1.7g, Saturated Fat: 0.8g, Unsaturated Fat: 0.9g, Potassium: 78.3mg, Protein: 5.3g, Sodium: 251.3mg, Dietary Exchanges: 1 Starch, 1/4 Very Lean Meat.

APRICOT BREAKFAST MUFFINS

1 cup apple juice
1/2 cup dried apricots, chopped
1 3/4 cups plain flour
1/3 cup dry Cream of Wheat
1/3 cup sugar
2 tsp. low sodium baking powder
1/4 tsp. salt
1/8 tsp. nutmeg
1/4 cup margarine, melted
1 tsp. vanilla
3 egg whites, lightly beaten
8 oz. plain nonfat yogurt
cooking spray
2 Tbsp. sugar

Preheat oven to 400 degrees. Bring apple juice and apricots to boil in a small saucepan over medium heat. Boil 1 minute then remove from heat and cover until cool. Strain over a bowl and save the juice. In a mixing bowl, combine the dry Cream of Wheat, flour, sugar, baking powder, salt, and nutmeg. Whisk together in a small bowl, 3 Tbsp. of the cooled juice, melted margarine, vanilla, egg whites, and yogurt. Gradually stir in the dry mixture. Stir in apricots. Coat a muffin pan with cooking spray. Divide the batter into the 12 muffin cups. Bake at 400 degrees for about 20 minutes, or until done. Cool on a wire rack. Dip the cooled muffins in the reserved apple juice in the saucepan and sprinkle with the 2 Tbsp. sugar. (DO NOT add any more sugar! The 2 Tbsp. should be lightly used for all 12 muffins!) Makes 12 servings.

Calories: 174.2, Total Carbs: 30.8g, Dietary Fiber: 1.1g, Sugars: 12.3g, Total Fat: 4.1g, Saturated Fat: 0.8g, Unsaturated Fat: 3.3g, Potassium: 187.6mg, Protein: 4.5g, Sodium: 80.2mg, Dietary Exchanges: 1 Fat, 1/4 Fruit, 1/4 Other Carbohydrates, 1 Starch.

Sharon Fox

ASPARAGUS QUICHE

3 Tbsp. margarine, melted
24 unsalted crackers (unsalted "Saltines"), crushed
1 1/2 cups evaporated skim milk
1 cup liquid egg substitute
1 tsp. dry mustard
1 tsp. Worcestershire sauce
1/8 tsp. nutmeg
1 pinch black pepper
1 lb. fresh asparagus, trimmed to 1 1/2 inch pieces

Preheat oven to 350 degrees. Combine the melted margarine and crushed crackers. Press the mixture into the bottom and up the sides of a 10 inch pie plate. Bake for 5 minutes to set the crust. Set aside.
Combine the milk, egg substitute, dry mustard, Worcestershire, nutmeg, and pepper. Stir in asparagus. Pour into the crust and bake 30-35 minutes until set. Allow to stand for 10 minutes before cutting. Makes 6 servings.

You can also bake these in 6 little tart pans so everyone will have their own little quiche!

Calories: 134.5, Total Carbs: 14.2g, Dietary Fiber: 2.5g, Sugars: 3.5g, Total Fat 6.9g, Saturated Fat: 1.4g, Unsaturated Fat: 5.5g, Potassium: 220mg, Protein: 3.8g, Sodium: 160.1mg, Dietary Exchanges: 1 1/4 Fat, 1/2 Starch, 1 Vegetable.

BANANA FRENCH TOAST POCKETS

cooking spray
2 eggs
1/2 cup fat-free milk
1/2 tsp. vanilla
1/8 tsp. cinnamon
4 pieces French bread, sliced in 1-inch thick slices
2/3 cup banana, thinly sliced
1 Tbsp. sifted powdered sugar

Preheat oven to 350 degrees. Line a baking sheet with aluminum foil and spray with cooking spray. In a shallow bowl combine eggs, milk, vanilla, and cinnamon. Whisk until well blended. Using a knife, cut a pocket into the side of each slice of bread, starting at the top crust.

Fill pockets with banana slices. Dip bread slices in egg mixture. Lay them on the prepared baking pan. Bake for 12 minutes until golden brown, turning once. Serve with powdered sugar or a LIGHT pancake syrup product or maple syrup. makes 4 servings.

Calories: 164.1, Total Carbs: 25.7g, Dietary Fiber: 1.5g, Sugars: 5.6g, Total Fat: 3.2g, Saturated Fat: 1g, Unsaturated Fat: 2.2g, Potassium: 165.1mg, Protein: 8.3g, Sodium: 259.6mg, Dietary Exchanges: 1/4 Fruit, 1/2 Meat, 1 1/4 Starch

BERRY BREAKFAST BARS

cooking spray
16 oz. fresh or frozen blackberries (or raspberries)
2 1/2 Tbsp. cornstarch
1 Tbsp. fresh lemon juice
1 cup unbleached white flour
1 cup whole wheat flour
2 cups quick cooking rolled oats
1 cup brown sugar
1 1/4 tsp. low sodium baking powder
3/4 tsp. ground allspice
1 tsp. cinnamon
1 cup unsalted butter or margarine

Preheat oven to 400 degrees. Spray a 9x13x2 inch baking pan with cooking spray. Thaw berries if you're using frozen ones. Warm the berries in a saucepan until the juices begin to run out. Reserve 1 cup of the juice, adding some water if needed, to make 1 cup. Cool the juice. Combine the cooled juice with cornstarch and lemon juice. Cook and stir until thickened. Gently stir in the berries. Set aside.

In a mixing bowl, combine the flour, oats, brown sugar, baking powder, salt, and spices. Cut in the butter until crumbly. Press 2/3 of the mixture into the prepared baking pan. Bake 15 minutes until lightly browned. Cool slightly. Spread the berries over the crust. Crumble the remaining mixture over the top of the berry mixture. Press slightly. Bake 20-25 minutes until the top is lightly browned. Cool completely in the pan. Cut into 24 bars. Makes 8 servings.

Calories: 20.6, Total Carbs: 1.5g, Dietary Fiber: 0.4g, Sugars: 0.9g, Total Fat: 1.5g, Saturated Fat: 0.1g, Unsaturated Fat: 1.4g, Potassium: 21.2mg, Protein: 0.6g, Sodium: 0.2mg, Dietary Exchanges: 1/4 Fat.

MORNIN' BREAKFAST WRAPS

cooking spray
2 eggs (or liquid substitute to equal 2 eggs)
1/8 tsp. black pepper
4 whole wheat tortillas
1 cup shredded frozen hash browns
1/2 of a green bell pepper, diced
1 oz. Canadian bacon, chopped
1/8 tsp. black pepper
1 oz. fat-free shredded cheddar cheese

Preheat your oven to 350 degrees. Spray a small nonstick skillet with cooking spray and heat to medium low. Cook the eggs and black pepper to scramble eggs. Set aside. Wrap the tortillas in foil and warm in oven for 5 minutes.
Meanwhile in a medium bowl, stir together the potatoes, bell pepper, bacon, and 1/8 tsp. black pepper. Spray a small skillet with cooking spray and heat to medium high. Spread the potato mixture into skillet and cook 6-7 minutes on one side, or until the potatoes are light golden brown. Flip the mixture over and cook 5-6 minutes more.
To assemble the wraps, layer the ingredients across the middle of each tortilla with one-fourth of the scrambled eggs, potatoes, and cheese. Roll up and serve immediately. You may also wrap them in aluminum foil to reheat later. Makes 4.

Calories: 233.5, Total Carbs: 32.5g, Dietary Fiber: 2.8g, Sugars: 1.7g, Total Fat: 5.7g, Saturated Fat: 0.8g, Unsaturated Fat: 4.9g, Potassium: 44.6mg, Protein: 10.1g, Sodium: 301.3mg, Dietary Exchanges: 2 Starch, 1/4 Very Lean Meat.

BUTTERMILK BANANA BREAD

1 1/4 cup all purpose, unbleached flour
1/2 tsp. baking soda
1/4 tsp. salt
1 large egg
1/3 cup honey
2 Tbsp. canola oil
1/4 cup low-fat buttermilk
1 cup sliced fresh bananas, mashed
1/4 cup raisins
1/4 cup chopped walnuts
cooking spray

Preheat oven to 350 degrees. In a small bowl, combine the flour, baking soda, and salt. Using an electric mixer, beat the honey, egg, and oil in a large bowl until smooth. Add half of the flour mixture and continue mixing on medium speed. Beat in the buttermilk and then add the rest of the flour mixture. Mix well. Add the mashed banana. Stir in the raisins and walnuts.

Pour batter into a 9x5 inch loaf pan, that has been sprayed with cooking spray, for 50 minutes, or until a toothpick inserted comes out clean. Turn the loaf out onto a wire rack to cool completely. Makes 16 servings.

Calories: 79.3, Total Carbs: 11.2g, Dietary Fiber: 0.6g, Sugars: 3.2g, Total Fat: 3.3g, Saturated Fat: 0.4g, Unsaturated Fat: 2.9g, Potassium: 51.9mg, Protein: 1.9g, Sodium: 83.9mg, Dietary Exchanges: 1/2 Fat, 1/4 Other Carbohydrates, 1/2 Starch.

CHAI HOT CHOCOLATE

1/2 cup fat-free milk
1/2 cup cold water
1 spiced Chai tea bag
1 packet dry (fat-free) hot chocolate mix

Heat milk and water to boiling then pour into mug. Add tea bag, let stand for at least 1 minute. Remove tea bag and stir in the hot chocolate mix. Makes one serving.

Calories: 70, Total Carbs: 11.5, Dietary Fiber: 0.8g, Sugars: 9g, Total Fat: 0g, Saturated Fat: 0g, Unsaturated Fat: 0g, Potassium: 190mg, Protein: 6.5g, Sodium: 199.7mg, Dietary Exchanges: 1/2 Milk, 1/4 Other Carbohydrates

CHALLAH FRENCH TOAST WITH FRESH BERRIES

2 eggs, beaten (or 1/2 cup Egg Beaters)
2 tsp. fat-free milk
4 slices Challah (egg bread)
1 tsp. canola oil
1 pinch cinnamon (for garnish)
2 cups fresh strawberries, sliced

Whisk together the egg and milk. Dip sliced bread into the egg mixture. Heat oil in skillet over medium heat. Place coated bread slices in heated skillet and brown on both sides. Put one slice one each plate. Garnish with cinnamon topped with sliced berries. Makes 4 servings.

Calories: 186.8, Total Carbs: 25.8g, Dietary Fiber: 2.6g, Sugars: 5.1g, Total Fat: 6.3g, Saturated Fat: 1.5g, Unsaturated Fat: 4.8g, Potassium: 206.6mg, Protein: 7.6g, Sodium: 234mg, Dietary Exchanges: 1/2 Fat, 1/2 Fruit, 1/2 Meat, 1 1/4 Starch.

SAUSAGE AND CHEDDAR CHEESE QUICHE

cooking spray
8 oz. fresh mushrooms, sliced
1/2 cup onion, chopped
12 oz. breakfast sausage
4 eggs
8 egg whites
1/4 cup shredded cheddar cheese
1/2 cup whole milk
1/4 tsp. salt
1/4 tsp. black pepper

Preheat oven to 350 degrees. Lightly coat skillet with cooking spray and heat over medium heat. Add mushrooms and onions. Cook, stirring occasionally, until onions are soft, about 8 minutes. Put the cooked onions and mushrooms into a mixing bowl. In a separate bowl, lightly beat the eggs and set aside. In another bowl, lightly beat the egg whites and set aside. Place the sausage in skillet and cook until done. Crumble and drain on paper towels. Combine the sausage, eggs, egg whites, cheese, milk, salt, and pepper with mushroom mixture in bowl. Lightly coat a 10 inch pie plate with cooking spray. Spoon the mixture into the pie plate. Bake for 30 minutes, until completely set. Allow to rest for 5 minutes before cutting. Cut into 8 slices and serve warm. This is a great dish to serve for brunch!
Makes 8 servings.

Calories: 252.2, Total Carbs: 2.9g, Dietary Fiber: 0.4g, Sugars: 1.9g, Total Fat: 20.1g, Saturated Fat: 6.8g, Unsaturated Fat: 13.3g, Potassium: 262.3mg, Protein: 14.8g, Sodium: 480.4mg, Dietary Exchanges: 3 Fat: 1 Meat, 1/4 Vegetable, 1/2 Very Lean Meat

CHOCOLATE CHERRY BREAKFAST SMOOTHIE

3/4 cup frozen, unsweetened sour red cherries
4 oz. sugar-free, fat-free vanilla yogurt
1/4 cup fat-free milk
1 Tbsp. cocoa powder
4 ice cubes
1 tsp. honey

Combine yogurt, milk, cocoa, frozen cherries, and ice in a blender. Blend on high setting for 30-60 seconds. Stir in the honey. Serve immediately. Makes 1 serving, 12 oz.

Calories: 155.9, Total Carbs: 29.6g, Dietary Fiber: 29.6g, Sugars: 21g, Total Fat: 1g, Saturated Fat: 0.1g, Unsaturated Fat: 0.9g, Potassium: 324.8mg, Protein: 7.8g, Sodium: 101.2mg, Dietary Exchanges: 1 Fruit, 1 Milk.

EASY CINNAMON WAFFLES AND BERRIES

3/4 cup unsweetened frozen blueberries
1 1/2 cups frozen unsweetened strawberries, cut into quarters
1/2 tsp. cinnamon
1/8 tsp. ground cloves
2 Tbsp. dark brown sugar, packed
1/4 tsp. almond extract
8 frozen whole wheat waffles

Put all the berries in a strainer and run under cold water to thaw. Set aside on a paper towel.

Place all ingredients except the waffles into a bowl and carefully combine. Let sit for 10 minutes. Toast the waffles and serve with the berries on top. Makes 8 servings.

For an added treat, serve with 1/3 cup low-fat vanilla yogurt!

Calories: 161.7, Total Carbs: 25.2g, Dietary Fiber: 3.6g, Sugars: 10.4g, Total Fat: 4.8g, Saturated Fat: 0.5g, Unsaturated Fat: 4.3g, Potassium: 83.1mg, Protein: 2.7g, Sodium: 211.6mg, Dietary Exchanges: 1 Fat, 1/2 Fruit, 1 Starch.

GRANNY'S CINNAMON OATMEAL WITH RAISINS

1/2 cup cold water
1/4 tsp. salt
2 Tbsp. seedless raisins
2/3 cup quick-cooking rolled oats
1 tsp. ground cinnamon

In a small saucepan combine the water, salt, and raisins. Bring to a boil. Stir in the oats and cinnamon, then reduce heat and simmer for 1 minute or until the water has absorbed. Remove from heat and serve warm.

My grandson, Exodus loves this!

When included in your diet regularly, oatmeal is a great way to help reduce your cholesterol. For a slightly different but equally delicious taste, try using Craisins (dried cranberries) or blueberries in place of the raisins!

Calories: 57, Total Carbs: 10.1g, Dietary Fiber: 1.8g, Sugars: 0.5g, Total Fat: 1g, Saturated Fat: 0g, Unsaturated Fat: 1g, Potassium: 2.9mg, Protein: 2.9mg, Protein: 2g, Sodium: 149mg, Dietary Exchanges: 1/4 Fruit, 1 Starch

CINNAMON AND SPICE FRUIT

1 medium orange
1 can (15.25 oz) canned pineapple chunks in water, (don't drain)
32 oz. canned pears in water, drained
16 oz. canned apricot halves with skin, drained
2 cinnamon sticks
6 whole cloves

Reserving the rind, peel the orange, section it and remove the seeds. Drain the pineapple and reserve the juice. In a large bowl, combine the orange sections, pineapple chunks, pear halves, and apricot halves. Set aside. In a saucepan, combine the orange rind, pineapple juice, cinnamon sticks, and cloves. Bring to a boil, reduce heat, then simmer for 5 minutes. Remove from heat. Strain the mixture and discard the rind and the whole cloves and cinnamon sticks. Pour the juice over the fruit and toss gently to coat. Cover and refrigerate to chill thoroughly. Makes 8 servings for breakfast or between meal snacks!

Calories: 117.7, Total Carbs: 30.5g, Dietary Fiber: 6.4g, Sugars 23.6g, Total Fat: 0.3g, Saturated Fat: 0g, Unsaturated Fat: 0.3g, Potassium: 354.7mg, Protein: 1.9g, Sodium: 7.4mg, Dietary Exchanges: 2 Fruit.

DELICIOUS COTTAGE CHEESE PARFAITS

1 cup unsweetened applesauce
2 cups fat-free cottage cheese
11 oz. canned mandarin oranges, drained
1/4 tsp. ground nutmeg

Layer 1/4 of each of the first 3 ingredients in the listed order in 4 parfait glasses. Top each with a pinch of nutmeg. Makes 4 servings.
This is a terrific breakfast or dessert treat!

Calories: 162.9, Total Carbs: 28.8g, Dietary Fiber: 2.5g, Sugars: 23.9g, Total Fat: 0.1g, Saturated Fat: 0g, Unsaturated Fat: 0.1g, Potassium: 223.7mg, Protein: 13.2g, Sodium: 468.6mg, Dietary Exchanges: 1 1/4 Fruit, 2 Very Lean Meat.

CRAB CASSEROLE

1 Tbsp. canola oil
12 eggs
1/2 cup fat-free milk
1 tsp. salt
1/2 tsp. white pepper
1 1/2 tsp. fresh dill weed, chopped
8 oz. cooked crab
8 oz. low-fat cream cheese, cubed
2 green onions, chopped
pinch of paprika

Pour oil into 8x8x2-inch square baking dish. Coat the dish evenly. In a large bowl, beat eggs, milk, salt, white pepper, and dill weed with a fork or wire whisk until well blended. Stir in crab meat, cream cheese, and onions. Pour into baking dish. Cover and refrigerate at least 4 hours, but no longer than 24 hours.

Heat oven to 35o degrees. Sprinkle paprika over the mixture. Bake 45-50 minutes or until the center is set. Makes 8 servings.

Great for breakfast or brunch!

Calories: 174, Total Carbs: 2.1g, Dietary Fiber: 0.1g, Sugars: 1.4g, Total Fat 10.3g, Saturated Fat: 2.9g, Unsaturated Fat: 7.4g, Potassium: 220.8mg, Protein: 17.4g, Sodium: 529.8mg, Dietary Exchanges: 1 Fat, 1 Very Lean Meat.

EGG WHITE OMLET

1/2 cup fresh broccoli, chopped (or thawed if frozen)
1/4 cup chopped red onion
1 clove garlic, minced
3/4 cup fresh spinach
4 egg whites
1/8 tsp. black pepper
1/2 cup reduced fat, shredded cheddar cheese
1 pinch salt
3 Tbsp. picante sauce

Spray medium nonstick skillet with olive oil spray. Set the pan over medium heat, adding the broccoli, onion, and garlic. Cook, stirring occasionally for 4-6 minutes, or until onion is almost tender. Add spinach, cooking 1-2 minutes until spinach is wilted. Remove the vegetables and set them on a plate, cover to keep them warm.

In a small bowl, whisk the egg whites and pepper. Coat the pan again with olive oil spray. Set over medium heat and pour egg white mixture into the pan. Cook, lifting the edges with a spatula as they begin to set and tipping the pan for uncooked egg whites to run underneath, for 2-3 minutes or until almost set. Flip over. Spoon the reserved vegetables over the egg white mixture. Sprinkle the cheese evenly over the top. Cover and cook for 1-2 minutes. Fold in half, move to serving plate, season with salt and pepper, and top with picante sauce. Serve immediately. Makes 2 servings.

Calories: 144.3, Total Carbs: 7.5g, Dietary Fiber: 1.9g, Sugars: 2.7g, Total Fat: 6.4g, Saturated Fat: 3.5g, Unsaturated Fat: 2.9g, Potassium 236mg, Protein: 15.4g, Sodium: 593.2mg, Dietary Exchanges: 1 Meat, 1 Vegetable, 1 Very Lean Meat

SPANISH OMLET

2 Tbsp. olive oil
1 medium onion, chopped
2 medium cloves garlic, crushed
2 small zucchini, thinly sliced
1 large potato, peeled
4 oz. fresh green beans, trimmed
2 eggs
2 egg whites
1/2 tsp. salt
1 pinch black pepper
1 large tomato, peeled, seeded, and chopped
1/2 tsp. dried oregano (or 2 Tbsp. fresh oregano)

In a heavy frying pan over medium heat, heat 1 1/2 Tbsp. of the oil. Add the onion and cook it for about 2-3 minutes, until soft. Add the garlic and zucchini, cover the pan and continue cooking gently for about 10 minutes. Stir occasionally and remove from heat once it's done.

In a small saucepan, boil the potato until tender, about 25 minutes. Remove the potato and add the green beans to the same water, cooking until tender. Chop the potato. Cut the green beans into 1-inch pieces. In a large bowl, beat eggs, egg whites, salt, and some black pepper. Stir in the cooked veggies, tomato, and oregano. In a nonstick 10-inch oven-proof skillet, heat the remaining oil and pour in the egg mixture. Cook over medium heat for 3-4 minutes, or just until the underside is pale gold. Place the pan under a preheated broiler and cook for 2-3 minutes, or until just set. Cut into squares and serve immediately. Makes 4 servings.

Eliminating the egg yolks in this recipe cuts a large amount of fat and cholesterol that you find in traditional omlets!

Calories: 222.9, Total Carbs: 26.6g, Dietary Fiber: 4.2g, Sugars: 5.8g, Total Fat: 9.9g, Saturated Fat: 1.8g, Unsaturated Fat: 8.1g, Potassium: 405.5mg, Protein: 8.9g, Sodium: 369.5mg, Dietary Exchanges: 1 1/2 Fat, 1/2 Meat, 1 Starch, 2 Vegetable.

FROSTY FRUITY SMOOTHIES

1 medium banana, cut into chunks
1 cup chilled juice; pineapple, orange, apple, grape, or low-cal cranberry)
1/2 cup fat-free milk
1 tsp. vanilla extract
3 ice cubes

Combine banana chunks, chilled fruit juice, milk, vanilla, and ice cubes in a blender. Cover and blend until frothy. Divide equally between two chilled glasses. Enjoy! Makes 2 servings.

Calories: 138.7, Total Carbs: 30g, Dietary Fiber: 2.5g, Sugars: 25.3g, Total Fat: 0g, Saturated Fat: 0g, Unsaturated Fat: 0g, Potassium: 183.2mg, Protein: 4.3g, Sodium: 157.7mg, Dietary Exchanges: 2 Fruit, 1/4 Milk.

GRANOLA FRENCH TOAST

2 egg whites, lightly beaten
2/3 cup low fat milk
1 tsp. orange zest
1 tsp. vanilla
1 cup granola, crushed
1 Tbsp. unsalted butter
8 slices whole wheat bread

Mix together the egg whites, milk, orange zest, and vanilla. Put the granola in a separate bowl. Place each slice of bread into the egg mixture, and then into the granola. Melt one-fourth of the butter on a griddle or in a large skillet. Place 2 prepared bread slices on hot griddle/skillet and cook each side for about 3 minutes or until golden brown. Continue the same steps with remaining bread until all have been cooked. Makes 4 servings.

Try adding sliced bananas on top. Great with maple syrup or syrup product. Watch your intake!

Calories: 263.3, Total Carbs: 35.7g, Dietary Fiber: 5.4g, Sugars: 8.4g, Total Fat: 7.6g, Saturated Fat: 2.4g, Unsaturated Fat: 5.2g, Potassium: 168.4mg, Protein: 12.6g, Sodium 323.8mg, Dietary Exchanges: 1/2 Fat, 2 1/4 Starch.

SWEET POTATO BISCUITS

15 oz. can yams, drained and mashed
4 cups Bisquick baking mix
1/2 tsp. cinnamon
1/4 cup fat free milk
3 Tbsp. 80% fat unsalted margarine, softened

Preheat your oven to 450 degrees. Use a mixing bowl and combine the mashed yams with cinnamon and baking mix. Add the milk and margarine and stir until blended. Roll onto a floured surface to about 1-inch thick. Cut with a 2-inch diameter biscuit cutter (or a drinking glass!). Place on ungreased baking sheet. Bake for 10-12 minutes or until golden brown. Makes 20 servings.

Calories: 72.4, Total Carbs: 11.7g, Dietary Fiber: 0.9g, Sugars: 2.7g, Total Fat: 2.4g, Saturated Fat: 0.5g, Unsaturated Fat: 1.9g, Potassium: 140mg, Protein: 1.2g, Sodium: 75.3mg, Dietary Exchanges: 1/2 Fat, 1 Starch.

NOTES

NOTES

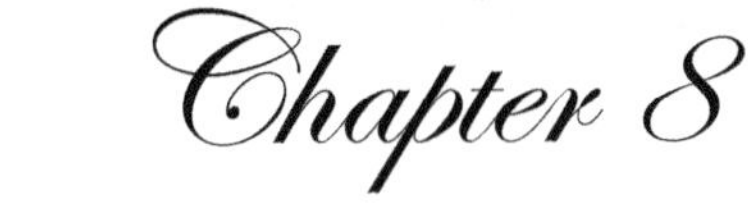

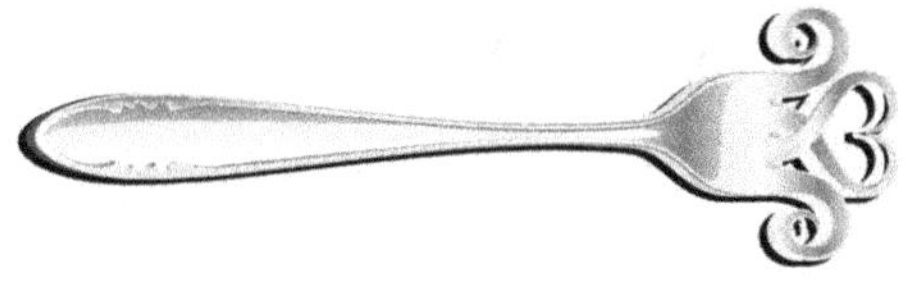

~DIABETIC LUNCH & SNACK~

HEALTHY CHICKEN ALMOND SALAD

8 oz. boneless, skinless chicken breasts, cooked and cut into strips
2 stalks celery, sliced
1 Tbsp. slivered almonds
2 Tbsp. fat-free mayonnaise
1 tsp. dried dill
pinch of salt
pinch of black pepper

Chop the cooked chicken strips and celery and put it in a mixing bowl. Toast almonds in a dry skillet over medium heat or in the oven, just until you smell the toasty aroma, lightly golden in color. Add toasted almonds to the chicken and celery. Stir in remaining ingredients. Spoon salad onto 2 plates and serve with a slice of rye bread or on top of a large lettuce leaf.
Makes 2 servings.

Calories: 169, Total Carbs: 5g, Dietary Fiber: 1.5g, Sugars: 1.1g, Total Fat: 2.4g, Saturated Fat: 0.5g, Unsaturated Fat: 1.9g, Potassium: 371.8mg, Protein: 30.5g, Sodium: 254.6mg, Dietary Exchanges: 2 1/2 Meat, 1 Starch, 1/2 Vegetable, 4 Very Lean Meat.

ATL SANDWICH

2 Tbsp. light mayonnaise
4 slices whole wheat bread
4 leaves of Boston or Romaine lettuce
1 large tomato, thinly sliced
1 avocado, peeled and sliced
12 very thin slices of fresh cucumber
4 slices Swiss cheese

Lightly coat each slice of bread with light mayonnaise. Arrange 1 tomato slice, 1 avocado slice, 3 cucumber slices, and 1 slice of Swiss cheese on each slice of bread. Top each sandwich with one lettuce leaf. Slice in half diagonally. Serve as open faced or place one half on top of the other. Makes 4 servings.

Calories: 280.6, Total Carbs 19.8g, Dietary Fiber: 4.2g, Sugar: 3.6g, Total Fat: 17.1g, Saturated Fat: 6.2g, Unsaturated Fat: 10.9g, Potassium: 444.4mg, Protein: 14.9g, Sodium: 255mg, Dietary Exchanges: 3 Fat, 1 1/4 Meat, 1 Starch, 1/2 Vegetable.

APRICOT-YOGURT SNACK

1/4 cup low-sugar apricot preserves
8 oz. sugar-free apricot-mango yogurt
2 tsp. Stevia (or your favorite sugar substitute)

Whisk the preserves in a bowl to loosen. Stir in the yogurt and sugar substitute until well blended. Spoon into small dessert bowls and serve. You can use any flavor yogurt to make it a fruit combination. Makes 2 servings.

Calories: 116, Total Carbs: 28.5g, Dietary Fiber: 0g, Sugars 23.2g, Total Fat: 0g, Saturated Fat: 0g, Unsaturated Fat: 0g, Potassium: 166.8mg, Protein: 3.3g, Sodium: 56.7mg, Dietary Exchanges: 1 Milk, 1 Other Carbohydrate.

GUACAMOLE CHICKEN SOUP

9 cups low-sodium chicken broth (or vegetable broth)
2 fresh avocados
pinch of salt
2 Roma tomatoes
2 whole jalapeno peppers
1/4 cup fresh cilantro, minced
1 Tbsp. fresh lime juice
1 tsp. lime zest

In a large saucepan over medium-high heat, bring the broth to a boil. Turn down heat and simmer 10 minutes.

While the broth is heating, slice the peppers in half lengthwise, remove the seeds and mince the peppers. (Wear plastic gloves to protect your skin from the heat, do not rub your eyes!) Wash and dice tomatoes. Cut avocado in half, remove the pit, and scoop out the flesh. Place avocado in a small bowl. Add peppers, cilantro, tomatoes, lime juice, and salt to the avocado. Mash with a fork, leaving avocado slightly chunky. To serve, scoop a heaping tablespoon of the avocado mixture into each soup bowl. Ladle a cup of hot broth around the avocado mixture. Garnish with the lime zest and serve. Makes 8 servings.

Calories: 103.7, Total Carbs: 6.3g, Dietary Fiber: 3.7g, Sugars: 1.5g, Total Fat: 7.4g, Saturated Fat: 1.1g, Unsaturated Fat: 6.3g, Potassium: 522.4mg, Protein: 4.9g, Sodium: 628.3mg, Dietary Exchanges: 1 1/2 Fat.

FISH TACOS

1 tsp. vegetable oil
1/2 cup chopped chile pepper or bell pepper
1 leek, chopped
2 cloves garlic, crushed
pinch salt and pepper
1 cup chicken broth
2 large tomatoes, diced
1/2 tsp. ground cumin
1 1/2 lbs. halibut fillets
1 lime
12 corn tortillas or low-carb flour tortillas

Heat oil in a large skillet over medium heat. Saute the pepper, leek, and garlic until tender, add salt and pepper. Add the chicken broth and tomatoes to the mixture in the skillet, stir in cumin. Bring to a boil, reduce heat to low. Place the halibut into the mixture in the skillet, sprinkling with the lime juice. Cook 15-20 minutes or until the halibut flakes easily with a fork. Wrap portions in warm tortillas. Makes 12 servings.

*** To warm tortillas, roll in foil and place in 325 degree oven for 5 minutes.***
***** These tacos are great topped with cheese, guacamole, and shredded lettuce.***

Calories: 211, Total Carbs: 15.7g, Dietary Fiber: 2.4g, Sugars: 1.5g, Total Fat: 4g, Saturated Fat: 0.4g, Unsaturated Fat: 3.6g, Potassium: 380.8mg, Protein: 26.4g, Sodium: 188mg, Dietary Exchanges: 3/4 Starch, 1/2 Vegetable, 3 1/2 Very Lean Meat.

TUNA MAC AND CHEESE CASSEROLE

10 3/4 oz. low-sodium cream of mushroom, ready to serve soup
1/3 cup fat-free milk
1 tsp. dried parsley
1/8 tsp. black pepper
1 cup plus 2 Tbsp. reduced fat mild cheddar cheese, shredded
2 cups cooked macaroni pasta, drained
6 oz. canned tuna, packed in water, drained
1/4 cup pimentos, drained and chopped
1/4 cup diced bell pepper
butter flavor cooking spray

Preheat oven to 375 degrees. Combine the soup, milk, parsley flakes, bell pepper, and black pepper in a skillet. Cook over low heat to soften the bell peppers. Stir in the cheddar and cook over medium heat until cheese melts, stirring often to prevent sticking. Stir in the cooked macaroni, tuna, and pimento before spreading into an 8x8-inch baking dish, sprayed with cooking spray. Bake for 20-25 minutes. Remove from oven and let stand 5 minutes before dividing into 4 equal servings.

Calories: 369.3, Total Carbs: 28.2g, Dietary Fiber: 2.3g, Sugars: 3.3g, Total Fat: 13.9g, Saturated Fat: 6.7g, Unsaturated Fat: 7.2g, Potassium: 225.7mg, Protein: 31g, Sodium: 278.5gm, Dietary Exchanges: 1 Fat, 1 1/4 Meat, 2 Starch, 2 1/2 Very Lean Meat.

BLUE CHEESE AND PEARS

1 1/2 oz. crumbled blue cheese
1/4 tsp. ground sage leaves, crumbled
1/4 of a garlic clove, minced
2 medium Bosc pears, halved
1 tsp. fresh lemon juice

Combine the cheese, sage, and garlic in a small bowl. Brush each side of pear halves with lemon juice just before serving. Fill each half with an equal amount of cheese mixture. Makes 4 servings.

Calories: 64.2, Total Carbs: 12.8g, Dietary Fiber: 2g, Sugars: 8.5g, Total Fat: 1.6g, Saturated Fat: 0.7g, Unsaturated Fat: 0.9g, Potassium: 10.8mg, Protein: 1.3g, Sodium: 50.1mg, Dietary Exchanges: 1 Fruit, 1/2 Meat.

BROWN PAPER BAG POPCORN

1/4 cup yellow popcorn, un-popped
pump butter spray
1/8 tsp. salt

Pour kernels into brown paper bag, fold closed to seal, and cook in microwave on the popcorn setting until the popping is complete. Remove from microwave, spray popcorn 10 times with butter spray, seal and shake. Repeat twice, add salt. Makes 4 servings.

Calories: 42.5, Total Carbs: 8.2g, Dietary Fiber: 1.8g, Sugars: 0.2g, Total Fat: 0.5g, Saturated Fat: 0g, Unsaturated Fat: 0.5g, Potassium: 32.5mg, Protein 1.2g, Sodium: 73.6mg, Dietary Exchanges: 1/2 Starch

DIVINE CAESAR SALAD

1 head fresh Romaine lettuce, shredded
2 Tbsp. grated Parmesan cheese
1 tsp. black pepper
2 Tbsp. fresh lemon juice
1 tsp. Worcestershire sauce
2 Tbsp. red wine vinegar
1/2 tsp. dry mustard
1/2 tsp. garlic powder
1/3 cup plain, whole milk yogurt
1 cup plain croutons, optional

In a large bowl, combine the lettuce, cheese, and black pepper. In a separate bowl, whisk together the lemon juice, Worcestershire sauce, vinegar, dry mustard, and garlic powder. Blend well. Add yogurt. Drizzle the dressing onto the lettuce and toss to coat. Add croutons, if desired. Makes 6 servings.

Calories: 31.7, Total Carbs: 3.3g, Dietary Fiber: 1.2g, Sugars: 1.4g, Total Fat: 1.4g, Saturated Fat: 0.8g, Unsaturated Fat: 0.6g, Potassium: 151mg, Protein: 2.2g, Sodium: 63.7mg, Dietary Exchanges: 1/4 Vegetable.

CRAB SALAD

2 1/4 cups cooked crab meat
3/4 cup canned artichoke hearts, drained and chopped
1/4 cup frozen green peas, thawed
3 Tbsp. chopped red onion
1/3 cup light mayonnaise
3 Tbsp. reduced-fat sour cream
1/8 tsp. ground thyme
pinch of white pepper

Toss the crab meat, artichoke hearts, peas, and onions together in a large bowl. In a small bowl, combine the mayonnaise, sour cream, thyme, and white pepper. Toss the mayonnaise mixture with the crab meat mixture, combining well. If it seems too dry, add a little more light mayonnaise. Cover and chill at least 2 hours before serving. Makes 4 servings.

*Use as a filling for a sandwich, serve in a cantaloupe half, or over a bed of fresh salad greens!

Calories: 262.9, Total Carbs: 8.1g, Dietary Fiber: 3.3g, Sugars: 2.8g, Total Fat: 9.5g, Saturated Fat: 1.9g, Unsaturated Fat: 7.6g, Potassium: 613.4mg, Protein: 32.8g, Sodium: 709.6mg, Dietary Exchanges: 1 1/2 Fat, Vegetable, 4 1/2 Very Lean Meat

CALIFORNIA WRAP

1 lettuce leaf
1 slice 95% fat-free oven-roasted white turkey deli meat
1 slice honey-baked ham deli meat
1 small tomato, sliced
1 slice of fresh avocado (1/5 of an avocado)
1 tsp. fresh lime juice
1 handful of fresh watercress or arugula greens
1 Tbsp. fat-free Ranch salad dressing

Open out the lettuce leaf on a plate. Top with turkey, ham, and tomato. In a small bowl, combine the avocado, lime juice, then spoon onto the tomato. Top with the watercress or arugula and Ranch dressing. Roll up and secure with a toothpick. Makes 1 serving.

Calories: 134.9, Total Carbs: 9.7g, Dietary Fiber: 4.4g, Sugars: 3.7g, Total Fat: 7.2g, Saturated Fat: 1.2g, Unsaturated Fat: 6g, Potassium: 276.6mg, Protein: 9.5g, Sodium: 402.4mg, Dietary Exchanges: 1 1/2 Fat, 1 Vegetable, 1 Very Lean Meat

Sharon Fox

BIG BATCH OF CANDY POPCORN

13 cups air popped popcorn
1 egg white
2 Tbsp. dark molasses
2 tsp. vanilla extract
1/2 tsp. salt
3/4 cup Stevia or Splenda (granulated)
1/2 cup dry roasted unsalted peanuts
cooking spray

Preheat oven to 325 degrees. Coat a 11x13 non-stick pan with cooking spray and set aside. In a large bowl, place popcorn and set aside. In a small bowl, whisk egg whites, molasses, vanilla, salt, and Stevia until well combined. Add the peanuts and stir until well-coated. Pour the egg mixture over the popcorn. Toss to coat the popcorn well. Place in the prepared baking pan and bake 20-25 minutes, stirring occasionally until crispy. Remove from oven and spread onto parchment or waxed paper to cool. When it reaches room temperature, it's ready to serve! Makes 10 servings.

*For a healthy treat, melt some dark chocolate and drizzle over cooled candy corn! Allow the chocolate to harden before serving.

Calories: 72.4, Total Carbs: 13.2g, Dietary Fiber: 1.7g, Sugars: 3.1g, Total Fat: 1.4g, Saturated Fat: 0.2g, Unsaturated Fat: 1.2g, Potassium: 128.9mg, Protein: 2.1g, Sodium: 124.8mg, Dietary Exchanges: 1/2 Starch

CANTALOUPE AND ROASTED STRAWBERRIES

1 cup fresh strawberries
1 Tbsp. powdered sugar (plus extra for dusting)
1/2 of a cantaloupe

Preheat broiler on high. Hull the berries and cut in half. Arrange them on a baking sheet in a single layer. Dust with 1 Tbsp. of powdered sugar. Broil the strawberries for 4-5 minutes or until the sugar begins to bubble and turn golden brown. Meanwhile, scoop out the seeds from the half melon and then remove the peel, using a sharp knife. Cut the melon into wedges and arrange them on a serving plate. Place the roasted strawberries on top. Dust with a little more powdered sugar, no more than 1 Tbsp. and serve immediately. Makes 4 servings.

Calories: 43.8, Total Carbs: 10.6g, Dietary Fiber: 1.2g, Sugars: 9.1g, Total Fat: 0.1g, Saturated Fat: 0g, Unsaturated Fat: 0.1g, Potassium: 55.1mg, Protein: 0.7g, Sodium: 12.9mg, Dietary Exchanges: 1/2 Fruit.

BANANAS AND CHEESECAKE SAUCE

1/2 cup fat-free sour cream
2 oz. low-fat cream cheese
7 tsp. fat-free milk
3 packets Splenda or Stevia
1/2 tsp. vanilla extract
pinch of nutmeg
3 bananas

Place the sour cream, cream cheese, milk, sugar substitute, and vanilla extract in a blender. Process until smooth. Pour 2 Tbsp. of the sauce into 6 individual plastic containers, sprinkle with nutmeg. Cover tightly and refrigerate until ready to serve. To serve, cut bananas in half and slice each half aside the 6 servings of sauce. Just dip a slice into sauce and enjoy! Makes 6 servings.

*If you want a tropical flavor, substitute coconut extract for the vanilla!

Calories: 81.7, Total Carbs: 18.9, Dietary Fiber: 1.5g, Sugars: 11.7g, Total Fat: 0.8g, Saturated Fat: 0.2g, Unsaturated Fat: 0.6g, Potassium: 2.9mg, Protein: 1.5g, Sodium: 33.7mg, Dietary Exchanges: 1 Fruit

CHEESY CHICKEN TACOS

6 oz. boneless skinless chicken breasts, trim, rinse and pat dry
olive oil cooking spray
3 Tbsp. minced onion
1 clove garlic, minced
1/4 tsp. chili powder
1/4 tsp. cumin
1/4 tsp. oregano
pinch of cayenne
pinch of salt and pepper
2 6-inch corn tortillas
1 cup shredded lettuce
2 Tbsp. reduced-fat shredded Monterey Jack cheese
1 Tbsp. cilantro, chopped
1/4 cup salsa
1/4 cup fat-free sour cream

Finely mince chicken. Preheat oven to 350 degrees. Spray a non-stick skillet with the cooking spray. Cook the onion and garlic over low heat until softened. Mix in the chicken, chili powder, cumin, oregano, cayenne, salt, and pepper. Cook and stir for about 5 minutes until chicken is done. Wrap tortillas in foil and place in oven for 5 minutes to warm them. Toss the cilantro and lettuce in a bowl. Set the tortillas on 2 plates, spoon the chicken mixture on them. Sprinkle with the lettuce mixture than add the sour cream and salsa to the top. Makes 2 servings.

Calories: 312.8, Total Carbs: 34.4g, Dietary Fiber: 2.5g, Sugars: 5.6g, Total Fat: 5.5g, Saturated Fat: 1.6g, Unsaturated Fat: 3.9g, Potassium: 403.7mg, Protein: 28.4g, Sodium: 312.1mg, Dietary Exchanges: 1/4 Meat, 1 1/4 Starch, 1 Vegetable, 3 Very Lean Meat

EEZY CHEEZY PRETZELS

1 1/2 cup all-purpose flour
1/2 cup sharp cheddar cheese, shredded
2/3 cup low-fat milk
2 Tbsp. margarine
2 tsp. low-sodium baking powder
1 tsp. sugar
1/2 tsp. salt
cooking spray
1 egg, beaten
pinch of coarse kosher salt

Preheat oven to 400 degrees. Spray cooking sheet with cooking spray and set aside. In a large bowl, combine all ingredients except the egg and kosher salt. Remove dough from the bowl and knead for 1-2 minutes on a lightly floured surface. Break dough into 12 balls (or 6 for large pretzels). Roll each ball into a thin rope and twist into pretzel knots or desired shapes. Place on a prepared cooking sheet. Brush with beaten egg and sprinkle with coarse salt. Bake 10-15 minutes or until browned. Makes 12 small or 6 large pretzels. 12 servings.

Calories: 105.8, Total Carbs: 13.5g, Dietary Fiber: 0.4g, Dietary Fiber: 0.4g, Sugars: 1g, Total Fat: 4.1g, Saturated Fat: 1.4g, Unsaturated Fat: 2.7g, Potassium: 106.5mg, Protein: 3.8g, Sodium: 165.8mg, Dietary Exchanges: 1/2 Fat, 1 Starch

SPINACH PIZZA

8 oz. frozen baby spinach, (in microwavable bag)
1/2 cup canned marinated artichoke hearts, drain, rinse, and chop
10 oz. thin, ready to heat pizza crust
1/2 cup part-skim shredded Mozzarella cheese
1/2 cup feta cheese, crumbled

Preheat broiler. Cook the spinach in the microwave according to package directions. Chop the spinach and place in a medium bowl. Stir in the artichokes. Place pizza crust onto a baking sheet and broil 4-5 inches from heat source until golden brown, about 30-60 seconds per side. Carefully remove the pan and leave the broiler on. Spread the spinach mixture over the crust leaving about 1-inch around the edges. Top with both cheeses. Broil until the mozzarella completely melts and the feta is partially melted, about 50-70 seconds. Cut into 6 slices. Makes 6 servings.

*If you prefer to cook your spinach on top of the stove, just add 1 Tbsp. water to it and cook about 2-3 minutes in a nonstick pan.

Calories: 213.4, Total Carbs: 29g, Dietary Fiber: 3.3g, Sugars: 0.9g, Total Fat: 6.5g, Saturated Fat: 2.4g, Unsaturated Fat 4.1g, Potassium 7.9mg, Protein: 10.2g, Sodium: 522.5mg, Dietary Exchanges: 1/4 Fat, 1/4 Meat, 1/2 Starch, 1 Vegetable

APRICOT-SWEET CHICKEN SALAD

2 lb. boneless, skinless chicken breast, cooked
8 oz. dried apricots, chopped
1/2 cup (1 bunch) chopped scallions
1/2 cup chopped celery
1/3 cup light mayonnaise
1/4 cup smooth honey-mustard
2 Tbsp. whole-grain honey-mustard
2 Tbsp. fresh lemon juice
2 Tbsp. fresh rosemary
1/3 cup sliced almonds, toasted

Shred the chicken with a fork into a large mixing bowl. Add the apricots, scallions, and celery. Stir to combine. In a small bowl, mix together the mayonnaise, both honey mustards, lemon juice, and rosemary. Combine the chicken mixture with the dressing mixture. Stir in toasted almonds. Refrigerate before serving. Makes 8 servings.

Calories: 288.7, Total Carbs: 21.9g, Dietary Fiber: 2.2g, Sugars, 2.6g, Total Fat: 6.9g, Saturated Fat: 1.1g, Unsaturated Fat: 5.8g, Potassium: 413.8mg, Protein: 31.5g, Sodium: 215.8mg, Dietary Exchanges: 1 Fat, 1 1/4 Fruit, 4 Very Lean Meat

CITRUSY ARUGULA SALAD

24 oz. canned pink grapefruit sections with juice
1 Tbsp. apple cider vinegar
2 tsp. Dijon mustard
1/2 tsp. salt
2 Tbsp. olive oil
10 oz. arugula (2 5oz. bags)
2 celery stalks, thinly sliced
1 medium yellow bell pepper, thinly sliced
1/3 cup golden raisins

Drain juice from the grapefruit, saving 1/4 cup for dressing. In a small bowl, whisk together the reserved grapefruit juice with cider vinegar, mustard, salt, and oil until well blended. Divide the arugula among 8 salad plates. Top each with equal amounts of celery, yellow bell pepper, raisins, and grapefruit segments. Drizzle with the dressing and serve. Makes 8 servings.

Calories: 131.6, Total Carbs: 25g, Dietary Fiber: 1.6g, Sugars: 22.6g, Total Fat: 3.6g, Saturated Fat: 0.5g, Unsaturated Fat: 3.1g, Potassium: 394.9mg, Protein: 1.8g, Sodium: 203.5mg, Dietary Exchanges: 1 Fat, 1 1/2 Fruit, 1/4 Vegetable

GOBBLE-GOBBLE TURKEY NACHOS

olive oil cooking spray
20 baked tortilla chips
3 oz. 99% fat-free ground turkey
2 Tbsp. refried beans
1 Tbsp. nacho cheese sauce
2 Tbsp. salsa (drain if it's watery)
1 Tbsp. fat-free sour cream
1 tsp. fresh chives, chopped fine

Arrange chips in a medium size shallow bowl. Warm skillet over medium heat and spray with nonstick cooking spray. Add the turkey and cook, breaking into chunks, for 3-5 minutes until done. Reduce heat and stir in the refried beans. Meanwhile, spoon the cheese sauce into a microwavable bowl and heat in 15 second intervals until warm. Spoon the cooked turkey mixture over the chips. Drizzle with cheese sauce and spoon on the salsa and sour cream. Sprinkle chives over the top and serve immediately. Makes one delicious serving.

Calories: 191.5, Total Carbs: 14.4g, Dietary Fiber: 1.5g, Sugars: 2.3g, Total Fat: 4.1g, Saturated Fat: 0.7g, Unsaturated Fat: 3.4g, Potassium: 15.3mg, Protein: 24.4g, Sodium: 500.8mg, Dietary Exchanges: 1/2 Fat, 1 Starch, 1/2 Vegetable, 3 Very Lean Meat.

NOTES

NOTES

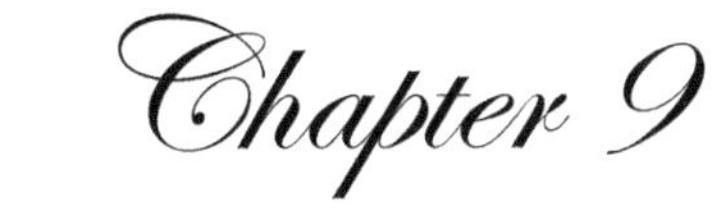

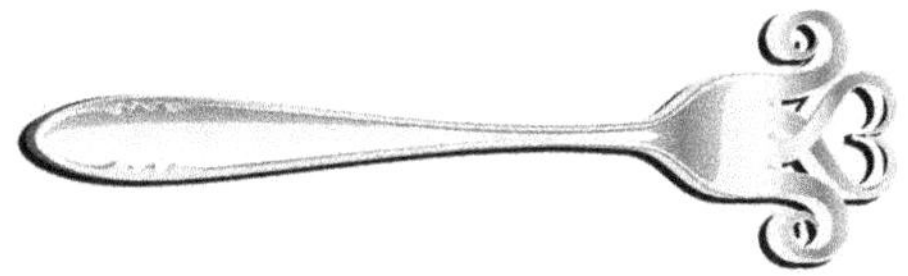

~DIABETIC MAIN DISHES~

GOURMET SIRLOIN STEAKS

1 lime, juiced
1 Tbsp. minced garlic
1 tsp. oregano
1 tsp. cumin
2 Tbsp. chipotle peppers in adobo sauce, chopped fine
4- 8oz. lean sirloin steaks
pinch of salt and pepper

In a small bowl, combine the lime juice, garlic, oregano, and cumin. Stir in the peppers and season to taste with the adobo sauce. Pierce the meat on both sides with a sharp knife, sprinkle with salt and pepper and place in a glass dish. pour the lime juice mixture over the meat and turn to coat both sides. Cover and allow it to marinate in the refrigerator about 2 hours. Preheat the grill (or skillet) to high. Lightly brush the grates with oil to prevent sticking. Place steaks on grill and cook for 6 minutes per side, or to desired doneness. Discard the marinade. Serve immediately. Makes 4 servings.

Calories 369.4, Total Carbs: 3.5g, Dietary Fiber: 1.1g, Sugars: 0.1g, Total Fat: 12.5g, Saturated Fat: 4.5g, Unsaturated Fat: 8g, Potassium 26.3mg, Protein: 56.2g, Sodium: 164mg. Dietary Exchanges: 1/2 Fat, 6 1/2 Meat, 8 Very Lean Meat.

BEEF STEW WITH OLIVES

2 lbs. beef chuck blade roast, trimmed
1 medium onion, chopped
1 medium tomato, chopped
2 garlic cloves, minced
2 bay leaves
2 cups unsalted, fat-free beef broth
2/3 cup cooking sherry
1/3 cup blanched whole almonds
1/2 cup pitted Calamata olives
1 tsp. cornstarch
2 Tbsp. chopped parsley

Cut beef into 1 inch cubes. Combine the beef, onion, tomato, garlic, bay leaves, and 1/3 cup water in a 6-qt. pot and bring to a boil over high heat. Cover, lower heat and continue to cook for 20 minutes. Remove lid, raise heat to medium. Continue to cook and stir frequently for 12-15 minutes. Allow the juices to evaporate and a dark film will form. Stir in the broth, 1/3 cup cooking sherry, and almonds. Scrape the brown film from sides and stir into sauce. Return to boil, cover and reduce heat to simmer. Allow to simmer for 1 hour. Stir in olives, place lid back on and simmer 15 more minutes. Meat should be tender. Continue to cook until liquid has reduced to 1 cup. Mix the remaining sherry with cornstarch and pour into the pot. Bring to boil and then remove from heat. Spoon into serving bowls and garnish with fresh chopped parsley on top. Makes 6 servings.

Calories: 360.3, Total Carbs: 9.5g, Dietary Fiber: 1.4g, Sugars: 2.8g, Total Fat: 17.7g, Saturated Fat: 5.2g, Unsaturated Fat: 12.5g, Potassium: 675mg, Protein: 35.7g, Sodium: 542.1mg, Dietary Exchanges: 1 Fat, 5 Meat, 1 Vegetable.

SIMPLE PORK CHOPS

4 boneless pork chops, about 3/4 inch thick
3/4 cup unsalted Italian Salad Dressing
1 tsp. low-sodium Worcestershire sauce

Place all ingredients in a good zip-lock bag. Seal and place in a dish in the refrigerator for 1 to 8 hours. Remove pork chops from bag, discard the marinade. Grill over medium heat about 5-6 minutes per side. Makes 4 servings.

Calories: 314.4, Total Carbs: 5.6g, Dietary Fiber: 0g, Sugars: 4g, Total Fat: 23.1g, Saturated Fat: 6g, Unsaturated Fat: 17.1g, Potassium: 365.8mg, Protein: 21.2g, Sodium: 438.1mg, Dietary Exchanges: 1/2 Fat, 3 Meat, 1/4 Other Carbohydrates.

APPLES AND CHICKEN

1/3 cup white whole wheat flour
1 tsp. salt (or to taste)
1/2 tsp. white pepper
2 tsp. garlic powder
2 tsp. ground sage
2 lbs. boneless, skinless chicken breasts
3 Tbsp. canola oil
4 medium Granny Smith apples, thinly sliced
2 cups apple cider
1 Tbsp. cornstarch
1 cup whole milk

Mix flour, salt, pepper, garlic powder, and sage in a shallow pan. Dredge the chicken in the flour mixture. Heat oil in a large skillet or Dutch oven over medium heat. Add chicken and brown each side for 5 minutes. In a large bowl, whisk together the cornstarch and milk. Stir in the apple cider. Add apple slices and cider mixture to the chicken. Simmer, uncovered until the apples are tender. This should take about 20 minutes. The cider should reduce by half during this time. Transfer to a serving platter. Serves 8.

Calories: 304, Total Carbs: 25.6g, Dietary Fiber: 3.4g, Sugars: 16g, Total Fat: 7.9g, Saturated Fat:: 1.4g, Unsaturated Fat: 6.5g, Potassium: 343.1mg, Protein: 31.5g, Sodium: 105.9mg, Dietary Exchanges: 1 Fat, 1 1/4 Fruit, 4 Very Lean Meat.

APRICOT AND MUSTARD PORK TENDERLOIN

1 lb. lean pork tenderloin
3 Tbsp. apricot preserves
1/4 cup Dijon mustard
1 pinch salt and pepper

Season the tenderloin with salt and pepper. Stir together the preserves and mustard in a small bowl. Place the meat over medium-high grill, or in 400 degree oven for about 15 minutes. Brush with mustard mixture and cook until done, about 3-5 minutes. Internal temperature should read 160 degrees. Makes 4 servings.

Calories: 190.3, Total Carbs: 12.7g, Dietary Fiber: 0g, Sugars: 9g, Total Fat: 3.4g, Saturated Fat: 1.2g, Unsaturated Fat: 2.2g, Potassium: 421.5mg, Protein: 25.2g, Sodium: 415mg, Dietary Exchanges: 2 1/2 Meat, 1/2 Other Carbohydrate.

ASIAN TUNA STEAKS

6- 4oz. tuna fillets

Marinade:
1/4 cup fresh orange juice
2 Tbsp. sesame oil
2 tsp. sesame seeds
3 Tbsp. low-sodium soy sauce
1 Tbsp. fresh grated ginger root
3 Tbsp. chopped scallions

Combine all marinade ingredients in a zip-lock bag or stainless steel bowl. Place tuna fillets in the marinade, coat evenly. Refrigerate for 20 minutes. Preheat the grill or skillet to medium heat. Cook 5 minutes on each side until done. Serve with some steamed vegetables! Makes 6 servings.

Calories: 242.6, Total Carbs: 2.3g, Dietary Fiber: 0.2g, Sugars: 1.3g, Total Fat: 11.5g, Saturated Fat: 2.3g, Unsaturated Fat: 9.2g, Potassium: 353mg, Protein: 30.8g, Sodium: 247.7mg, Dietary Exchanges: 2 Fat, 4 1/4 Very Lean Meat.

GREEK CHICKEN WITH LEMON SAUCE

4- 4oz. boneless, skinless chicken breasts
1 Tbsp. good olive oil
1/2 cup chopped onion
1/2 cup chopped green bell pepper
3/4 cup low-sodium chicken broth
2 Tbsp. fresh lemon juice
1 Tbsp. lemon zest
1 tsp. oregano
8 large canned black olives, sliced

In a large pan over medium heat, add oil. Heat to medium high and add the chicken. Cook for 5 minutes on each side, until brown. Add onion and bell pepper. Cook until the chicken is thoroughly cooked and vegetables are tender, about 5 more minutes.
In a small pot, add the broth, lemon juice, lemon zest, and oregano. Bring to a boil, reduce heat and cook for 5 minutes or until reduced to about 1/2 cup. Put the cooked chicken mixture onto serving plates. Top with sauce and sliced olives. Makes 4 servings.

Calories: 201.6, Total Carbs: 4.6g, Dietary Fiber: 1.3g, Sugars: 1.6g, Total Fat: 6.2g, Saturated Fat: 1.1g, Unsaturated Fat: 5.1g, Potassium: 443.7mg, Protein: 30.8g, Sodium: 265.8mg, Dietary Exchanges: 1 Fat, 1/2 Vegetable, 4 Very Lean Meat.

MINI BEEF WELLINGTONS

2 tsp. olive oil
1/2 lb. fresh mushrooms, finely chopped
3 Tbsp. dry red wine
3 Tbsp. chopped green onions
1/4 tsp. ground thyme
1/4 tsp. salt
1/8 tsp. pepper
1 lb. extra lean beef tenderloin, cut into 4 pieces
6 sheets frozen Phyllo pastry dough, thawed

Preheat oven to 425 degrees. Heat the oil in a large non-stick skillet over medium heat until hot. Add the mushrooms and cook, stirring for 5 minutes until tender. Add the wine and cook an additional 2-3 minutes or until the liquid evaporates. Stir in the green onions, thyme, salt, and pepper. Remove the skillet from heat and cool completely. Put the cooked mixture in a small bowl. Heat the same skillet over medium heat until hot. Place the steaks in skillet and cook 3 minutes, flipping only once. Steaks will only be partially cooked). Season with salt and pepper. Stack the pastry sheets on a flat surface, spraying each sheet with cooking spray. Cut the stacked sheets lengthwise in half, then crosswise to make 4 equal stacks. Place about 2 Tbsp. of the mushroom mixture in the center of each stack. Place the steaks on top of the mushroom mixture. Bring all 4 corners of the pastry together and twist tightly to close. Lightly spray each bundle with cooking spray and place on a greased baking sheet. Immediately bake at 425 degrees. for 9-10 minutes or until golden brown. Let stand 5 minutes. Serve immediately. Makes 4 servings.

Calories: 250.8, Total Carbs: 18g, Dietary Fiber: 1.1g, Sugars: 1.1g, Total Fat: 8g, Saturated Fat: 2.2g, Unsaturated Fat: 5.8g, Potassium: 280.6mg, Protein: 25.4g, Sodium: 197.4mg, Dietary Exchanges: 1 Fat, 2 1/4 Meat, 1 Other Carbohydrate, 1/2 Vegetable.

BAKED JAMAICAN CHICKEN WITH MANGO

2 whole jalapeno peppers, halved and seeded
1 medium onion, quartered
2 garlic cloves
1 Tbsp. fresh ginger root, minced
1 Tbsp. extra virgin olive oil
1 Tbsp. white wine vinegar
1 tsp. Caribbean jerk seasoning
1 tsp. ground allspice
1/4 tsp. salt
4 boneless, skinless chicken breasts
1/2 of a fresh mango, chopped finely
1 Tbsp. fresh cilantro, chopped
cooking spray

Preheat oven to 450 degrees. Coat a 9x13-inch baking pan with cooking spray. In a food processor or blender, combine peppers, onion, garlic, ginger, olive oil, vinegar, jerk seasoning, allspice, and salt. Process until very finely chopped. Spread this mixture on both sides of chicken breasts. Place coated chicken in prepared baking pan and bake for 30 minutes or until done. Place the cooked chicken on plates and scatter the chopped mango on top. Sprinkle with chopped cilantro. Makes 4 servings.

Calories: 192, Total Carbs: 7.3g, Dietary Fiber: 1.1g, Sugars: 1.8g, Total Fat: 5.4g, Saturated Fat: 0.9g, Unsaturated Fat: 4.5g, Potassium: 347.3mg, Protein: 26.5g, Sodium: 290.3mg, Dietary Exchanges: 1 Fat, 1/4 Fruit, 1/2 Vegetable, 3 1/2 Very Lean Meat.

OVEN BAKED FLOUNDER WITH DILL SAUCE

1- 8oz. flounder fillet
1 pinch salt
1 Tbsp. light mayonnaise
2 tsp. whole grain honey mustard
2 cloves garlic, minced
1 Tbsp. light soy sauce
2 Tbsp. fresh dill weed, chopped

Preheat oven to 375 degrees. Cut the fish into 2 inch slices and sprinkle with salt. Place in an oven-proof baking dish. Combine remaining ingredients and pour over fish. Cover and refrigerate for 2-3 hours, turning occasionally. Bake until fish is just done. Do not over-bake. Makes 4 servings.

Calories: 88, Total Carbs: 2.6g, Dietary Fiber: 0.1g, Sugars: 1.4g, Total Fat: 2.4g, Saturated Fat: 0.4g, Unsaturated Fat: 2g, Potassium: 339.3mg, Protein: 12.6g, Sodium: 254.5mg, Dietary Exchanges: 2 Very Lean Meat

BAKED SESAME CHICKEN

2 Tbsp. low-sodium soy sauce
1/4 cup toasted sesame seeds
2 Tbsp. all purpose flour
1/4 tsp. salt
pinch of black pepper
4 boneless, skinless chicken breasts
2 Tbsp. butter, melted

Preheat oven to 400 degrees. Place the soy sauce into a 9x13-inch baking dish. On a piece of wax paper, mix together the sesame seeds, flour, salt, and pepper. Dip the chicken into the soy sauce to coat and then roll them in sesame seed mixture. Arrange in a single layer in the same baking dish. Drizzle with melted butter. Bake for about 40 minutes or until the chicken is completely cooked through. Baste with drippings once during cooking. Makes 4 servings.

Calories: 244.5, Total Carbs: 4.8g, Dietary Fiber: 1g, Sugars: 0.1g, Total Fat: 11.3g, Saturated Fat: 4g, Unsaturated Fat: 7.3g, Potassium: 327.3mg, Protein: 29.1g, Sodium: 471.2mg, Dietary Exchanges: 2 Fat, 1/4 Starch, 4 Very Lean Meat.

BEEF BRISKET

5 lb. whole lean beef brisket, trimmed
pinch salt and pepper to taste
3 Tbsp. roasted garlic cloves, chopped
1/4 cup light honey
1/4 cup apple cider vinegar
1/4 cup light soy sauce
2 cups canned tomatoes, drained and chopped
2 Tbsp. dried Chipotle chili peppers, diced
1/4 cup fresh cilantro, chopped

Trim excess fat from brisket and season with salt and pepper. In a small bowl, combine the honey, vinegar, light soy, tomatoes, and chipotle pepper. Spread over brisket. Cover and refrigerate overnight. Preheat oven to 300 degrees. Transfer the brisket and marinade to Dutch oven or heavy baking dish. Bake covered 5-6 hours, or until tender. Sprinkle generously with finely chopped cilantro and serve. Makes 12 servings.

Calories: 367.8, Total Carbs: 7.9g, Dietary Fiber: 0.4g, Sugars: 7.1g, Total Fat: 15.9g, Saturated: 5.6g, Unsaturated Fat: 10.3g, Potassium: 721.1mg, Protein: 45.4g, Sodium: 434.4mg, Dietary Exchanges: 6 Meat, 1/4 Other Carbohydrate, 1/4 Vegetable.

BASIL-GARLIC STEAKS FOR TWO

1/2 tsp. olive oil
1 large garlic clove, mashed
1 8oz. lean strip steak or rib-eye, cut into two
3/4 cup white wine
3 fresh basil leaves, chopped
pinch of hot sauce, optional

Lightly cover the bottom of a cast iron skillet with olive oil. Gently heat the mashed garlic clove in it, just until aromatic and browning. Remove garlic and turn heat to high. Add the steaks and turn them briefly until browned. Add the wine, 1/4 cup at a time, allowing it to reduce completely between additions. Add the basil leaves. Remove steaks onto a warm serving plate after desired doneness has been reached. After 5-6 minutes they should be medium rare. Deglaze the skillet with1/2 cup of warm water to make a tasty light sauce. Add a little hot sauce if desired. Makes 2 servings.

Calories: 291.8, Total Carbs: 3.3g, Dietary Fiber: 0g, Sugars: 0.8g, Total Fat: 10g, Saturated Fat: 3.4g, Unsaturated Fat: 6.6g, Potassium: 78.9mg, Protein: 28.2g, Sodium: 69mg, Dietary Exchanges: 1 Fat, 3 1/2 Meat, 4 Very Lean Meat.

Sharon Fox

SUNDAY MEATLOAF

1/4 cup chopped onion
1/4 cup finely chopped celery
1/4 cup ketchup
2 egg whites
1/4 cup plain dry breadcrumbs
1 tsp. liquid smoke
1 tsp. salt
pinch black pepper
1 lb. extra lean ground beef, 95% lean

Preheat oven to 325 degrees. Place all ingredients EXCEPT beef into a bowl and mix together until well combined. Add ground beef and mix well. Shape into a loaf about 3 1/2" x 7" and place it on a baking pan sprayed with cooking spray. Bake for about 1 hour. Pour off all excess fat and let stand 10 minutes before serving. Makes 6 servings.

Calories: 123, Total Carbs: 6.8g, Dietary Fiber: 0.4g, Sugars: 3.3g, Total Fat: 2.9g, Saturated Fat: 1.1g, Unsaturated Fat: 1.8g, Potassium: 49.6mg, Protein: 17.9g, Sodium: 612.2mg, Dietary Exchanges: 1 1/2 Meat.

BEEF AND BLUE CHEESE CASSEROLE

cooking spray
12oz. extra lean ground beef (5% fat)
3 medium size onions, chopped
1 1/4 lbs. red potatoes, diced with skin left on
8 oz. fresh sliced mushrooms
1 cup cold water
2 tsp. low-sodium bouillon powder
1 tsp. dried oregano
1/2 tsp. black pepper
1/8 tsp. salt
1/2 cup crumbled blue cheese
1/4 cup chopped parsley

Spray a Dutch oven with vegetable cooking spray and heat over medium high heat. Add ground beef and cook until done, crumbling as it cooks. Place beef in a strainer and rinse under hot water to remove excess fat. Drain well and set aside. Wipe grease out of the Dutch oven with a paper towel and spray it again with cooking spray. Saute onions until softened. Add potatoes, mushrooms, water, beef bouillon, oregano, and pepper. Raise heat to high and bring to a boil. Lower heat to simmer, cover. Cook for about 10 minutes then remove from heat. Stir in cooked beef, salt, and blue cheese. Allow to sit for 2 minutes for the flavors to marry. Garnish with fresh parsley and serve. Makes 4 servings.

You could use ground turkey in place of beef.

Calories: 281.8, Total Carbs: 30.4g, Dietary fiber: 5.4g, Sugars: 8.5g, Total Fat: 7.5g, Saturated Fat: 3.7g, Unsaturated Fat: 3.8g, Potassium: 748.6mg, Protein: 25.5g, Sodium: 342mg, Dietary Exchanges: 2 Meat, 1 Starch, 2 Vegetable.

BEEF BOURGUIGNON (Slow-Cooker Method)

3 lbs. boneless top sirloin steak
1/2 cup whole wheat flour
4 slices bacon
4 small red potatoes, cut into quarters
1 cup fresh sliced mushrooms
2 medium carrots, sliced
2 cups pearl onions
3 cloves garlic, minced
1 bay leaf
1 tsp. marjoram
1/2 tsp. ground thyme
1/2 tsp. salt
1/4 tsp. black pepper
2 1/2 cups low-sodium beef broth or burgundy wine

Cut the steak into 1/2 inch pieces. Place flour in medium bowl, add beef. Toss to coat completely with flour. Remove from bowl, shaking off excess flour and set aside. In a large skillet over medium heat, cook bacon until partially done. Add beef to the skillet and brown on all sides. Remove the beef and bacon with a slotted spoon. In a slow cooker, layer the potatoes, mushrooms, carrots, onions, garlic, bay leaf, marjoram, thyme, salt, pepper, beef, and bacon. Add broth or wine and cover. Cook 8-10 hours on low setting until the beef is tender. Remove the bay leaf. Makes 12 servings.

Calories: 376.3, Total Carbs: 19.8g, Dietary Fiber: 2.3g, Sugars: 2.1g, Total Fat: 18.6g, Saturated Fat: 6.9g, Unsaturated Fat: 11.7g, Potassium: 341.1mg, Protein: 31.3g, Sodium: 154.6mg, Dietary Exchanges: 2 Fat, 4 Meat, 1 Starch, 1 Vegetable.

BEEF AND CHEESY SKILLET (BEEF-A-RONI)

2 cups macaroni (semolina) pasta
1 lb. extra lean ground beef (5% fat)
1 can (14.5oz.) can crushed tomatoes
8 oz. can tomato sauce
2 tsp. chili powder
dash of cayenne pepper
1 tsp. garlic powder
1 tsp. sugar substitute (I prefer Stevia)
2/3 cup low-fat cheddar cheese, shredded

Cook the pasta according to the directions on package. Drain. In a large skillet, cook the ground beef, drain any excess fat. Add remaining ingredients except cheese and pasta. Bring this mixture to a boil, reduce heat and simmer 5-7 minutes or until it begins to thicken. Stir in cheese and pasta. Makes 7 servings.

Calories: 239, Total Carbs: 20.5g, Dietary Fiber: 2.1g, Sugars: 2.8g, Total Fat: 5.9g, Saturated Fat: 2.8g, Unsaturated Fat: 3.1g, Potassium: 367.2mg, Protein: 27.8g, Sodium: 569.1mg, Dietary Exchanges: 1 1/4 Meat, 1 Starch, 1 1/4 Vegetable.

ROAST BEEF WITH MAPLE SWEET POTATOES

3 lbs. beef chuck roast, boned and trimmed of all fat
2 tsp. olive oil
1 3/4 tsp. salt, divided
3/4 tsp. black pepper, divided
1 cup chopped onion
2 tsp. fresh thyme, chopped
1 cup reduced sodium beef broth
3/4 cup apple cider
3 lbs. sweet potatoes, peeled and cut crosswise in 1 1/2-inch pieces
4 cloves garlic, peeled
2 Tbsp. maple syrup
1 tsp. minced ginger root
2 Tbsp. cornstarch
2 Tbsp. Brandy or water

Heat oil in a stockpot over medium heat until hot. Place the roast in the hot pot and brown evenly on all sides. Remove from pot and pour off drippings. Season with 1 tsp. salt and 1/2 tsp. pepper. Add onion and thyme to the pot. Cook and stir 5 minutes or until onion is tender. Add broth and cider. Turn heat up to medium-high. Cook 1-2 minutes until the little brown bits on the bottom of the pot are dissolved. Return the roast to the pot, bring to a boil. Reduce heat, cover with a tight-fitting lid and simmer 2 1/2 hours. Add the sweet potatoes and garlic and continue simmering until potatoes are fork-tender (about 30 minutes). Remove the roast, keep warm. Remove sweet potatoes and garlic with a slotted spoon to a large bowl, leave the cooking liquid in the pot. Add maple syrup, ginger, remaining 3/4 tsp. salt, and 1/4 tsp. pepper to the sweet potatoes. Beat until the sweet potatoes and garlic are mashed and smooth. Keep warm. Skim fat from cooking liquid. Dissolve the cornstarch in water or brandy. Stir into the cooking liquid. Bring to a boil, stir and cook until thickened. Carve the roast into slices. Serve with the mashed sweet potatoes and gravy. Makes 12 servings.

Calories: 357.9, Total Carbs: 36.8g, Dietary Fiber: 4.7g, Sugars: 10.4g, Total Fat: 9g, Saturated Fat: 2.8g, Unsaturated Fat: 6.2g, Potassium: 935.5mg, Protein: 29.1g, Sodium: 533.9mg, Dietary Exchanges: 3 1/4 Meat, 1 1/2 Starch, 1/4 Vegetable.

CABBAGE AU GRATIN

cooking spray
4 cups fresh cabbage, chopped
1 cup carrots, shredded
1/2 cup green onions, chopped
1 cup whole milk
1/4 cup gruyere cheese, shredded
1/2 tsp. caraway seeds
1/4 tsp. salt
2 eggs, lightly beaten
1 egg white
2 Tbsp. minced parsley
1 Tbsp. grated Parmesan cheese

Preheat your oven to 375 degrees. Coat a small saucepan with cooking spray and heat over medium heat. Add the cabbage, carrot, and onions. Cook until tender, about 5-7 minutes. Coat a 6x10- inch baking dish with cooking spray. Add the cabbage mixture to the baking dish. In a medium mixing bowl add the milk, cheese, caraway seeds, salt, eggs, and egg white. Stir to combine. Spoon the mixture over the cabbage and sprinkle with parsley and Parmesan cheese. Bake for about 35-40 minutes, or until a knife inserted in center comes out clean. Let rest 5 minutes before serving. Makes 6 servings.

*You can substitute different cheeses according to your taste.
**Try using different veggies in place of, or in addition to cabbage!

Calories: 100.5, Total Carbs: 7.9g, Dietary Fiber: 2.1g, Sugars: 5.3g, Total Fat: 5g, Saturated Fat: 2.5g, Unsaturated Fat: 2.5g, Potassium: 145.2mg, Protein: 6.9g, Sodium: 113.7mg, Dietary Exchanges: 1/4 Fat, 1 Vegetable

LAMB CHOPS WITH FETA CHEESE

1 1/2 oz. crumbled feta cheese
1 tsp. ground oregano
1/2 tsp. dried mint leaves, crumbled
1/2 tsp. minced garlic
4 3oz. boneless, lean lamb chops

Preheat broiler. Coat the rack of broiler pan with cooking spray. In a small bowl, combine feta cheese, oregano, mint, and garlic. Set aside. Broil the lamb chops on broiler rack 3-4 minutes until browned. Turn them over, spread the feta mixture over them and cook for 6-8 more minutes. Allow to rest 5 minutes before serving. Makes 4 servings.

Calories: 91.5, Total Carbs: 0.5g, Dietary Fiber: 0.1g, Sugars: 0.2g, Total Fat: 4.2g, Saturated Fat: 1.8g, Unsaturated Fat: 2.4g, Potassium: 158.8mg, Protein: 12.1g, Sodium: 82.5mg, Dietary Exchanges: 1 1/2 Meat

CREOLE PORK CHOPS WITH JASMINE RICE

2 tsp. salt-free Creole (Cajun) seasoning
3/4 tsp. no-sodium salt substitute
4 pork loin chops, about 1/4-inch thick, trimmed of all fat
cooking spray
1 cup jasmine rice
1 can (14.5oz) unsalted chicken broth
10oz. frozen green beans, thawed (or mixed vegetables)

Season the chops with 1 tsp. Creole seasoning and 1/2 tsp. salt substitute. Lightly spray a large nonstick skillet with cooking spray and heat over medium heat. Place chops in hot pan and cook until they are just about done, about 4 minutes on each side. Remove chops from pan and set aside. Add the rice, 1 tsp. Creole seasoning, 1/4 tsp. salt substitute, and broth to pan and bring to a boil. Lower heat to simmer, cover and cook 15 minutes. Add in the green beans, place chops on top. Cover and simmer until all the moisture is absorbed, about 8 minutes. Makes 4 servings.

Calories: 284.9, Total Carbs: 23.5g, Dietary Fiber: 2g, Sugars: 0g, Total Fat: 7.1g, Saturated Fat: 2.4g, Unsaturated Fat: 4.7g, Potassium: 996.9mg, Protein: 28.9g, Sodium: 417.9mg, Dietary Exchanges: 3 Meat, 1 Starch, 1 Vegetable.

BONUS: Make our own Salt-Free Cajun (Creole) Seasoning. Here's the recipe!

SALT-FREE CREOLE SEASONING

1 Tbsp. of EACH:
Chili powder, ground cumin, garlic powder, onion powder, and paprika.
Store in an airtight container. This will be good for about 6 months!

CARIBBEAN CHICKEN

4 boneless, skinless chicken breasts
2 tsp. fresh lime juice
1 tsp. vegetable oil
2 tsp. Caribbean jerk seasoning

Place the chicken breasts between two sheets of heavy plastic wrap. Flatten meat to 1/4-inch thick by using a mallet or rolling pin. In a small bowl, combine the lime juice and oil. Brush the mixture over both sides of meat and then rub the jerk seasoning all over it on both sides. Cook the chicken over medium-hot heat until done, about 5-6 minutes per side. Serve with rice and fresh fruits like papaya and mango! Makes 4 servings.

Calories: 135.4, Total Carbs: 0.2g, Dietary Fiber: 0g, Sugars: 0g, Total Fat: 2.5g, Saturated Fat: 0.5g, Unsaturated Fat: 2g, Potassium: 303.9mg, Protein: 26.2g, Sodium: 213.8mg, Dietary Exchanges: 3 1/2 Very Lean Meat.

TASTY CARNE GUISADA

1/2 Tbsp. all vegetable shortening
1 1/2 lbs. pork tenderloin, cubed
1 can (14.5oz) unsalted stewed tomatoes
2 jalapeno peppers, seeded and diced
2 tomatoes, chopped
1/2 tsp. cumin
1 garlic clove, minced
pinch of salt and pepper

Melt the shortening in a large saucepan over medium-high heat. Add the meat and brown well on all sides. Add the onions and saute for 5 minutes, until tender. Stir in the canned tomatoes, jalapeno peppers, fresh tomatoes, cumin, garlic, salt and pepper. Reduce heat to low for about 45 minutes to 1 hour, or until meat is tender. If the mixture is too thick, add a little water as needed. If it's too thin, combine some cornstarch mixed with a little water to make a thickener and stir into sauce. Makes 4 servings. Serve with wheat tortillas.

Calories: 289, Total Carbs: 13.1g, Dietary Fiber: 3.2g, Sugars: 8.7g, Total Fat: 6.1g, Saturated Fat: 1.9g, Unsaturated Fat: 4.2g, Potassium: 893.9mg, Protein: 42.1g, Sodium: 124.4mg, Dietary Exchanges: 1/4 Fat, 4 Meat, 4 Starch, 2 1/2 Vegetable, 5 Very Lean Meat.

CHICKEN FOR A KING

4 oz. can mushroom stems and pieces
2 Tbsp. vegetable oil
3 cups fat-free reduced sodium chicken broth
3 Tbsp. cornstarch
1/4 cup non-fat dry skim milk
1/8 tsp. white pepper
2 cups diced cooked chicken or turkey breast, skin removed
1/4 cup pimento, chopped

Pour oil into a saucepan. Drain the mushrooms, discard the juice, and add them to the saucepan. Cook until lightly browned, stirring occasionally. In a separate bowl, stir together the broth, cornstarch, dry milk, and pepper until smooth. Stir this mixture into the mushrooms and cook over medium heat until thickened. Stir in the cooked chicken cubes and pimento and heat through. Makes 4 servings. Serve over wheat toast or biscuit.

Calories: 218.5, Total Carbs: 9.1g, Dietary Fiber: 0.7g, Sugars: 2.8g, Total Fat: 9.9g, Saturated Fat: 1.8g, Unsaturated Fat: 8.1g, Potassium: 195.3mg, Protein: 22.1g, Sodium: 502.5mg, Dietary Exchanges: 1 1/2 Fat, 1/4 Vegetable, 3 Very Lean Meat.

HEALTHY CHICKEN AND KALE STUFFING

4 boneless, skinless chicken breasts
1 cup fresh sliced mushrooms
1/2 cup chopped onion
2 Tbsp. dry white wine
1/4 tsp. ground oregano, crushed
1 clove garlic, minced
1/2 tsp. black pepper
1 tsp. ground sage
2 cups chopped kale, washed
2 Tbsp. mayonnaise
1/2 cup seasoned whole wheat bread crumbs

Preheat your oven to 400 degrees. Coat a shallow baking dish with cooking spray and set aside. Trim all fat from chicken and pound it to 1/2 -inch thick and set aside. Heat large skillet over medium-high heat. Add mushrooms, onion, wine, oregano, sage, garlic, and pepper. Cook for about 5 minutes or until onions are softened. Add kale and cook until it wilts. Divide the mixture and spread on top of each flattened chicken breast. Roll up and secure with a toothpick or metal skewers. Brush the chicken with mayonnaise and coat with bread crumbs. Place chicken seam side down in the prepared baking dish. Bake for 25 minutes or until the chicken is golden brown and juices run clear. Remove toothpicks and serve. Makes 4 servings.

Calories: 269.4, Total Carbs: 16g, Dietary Fiber: 1.8g, Sugars: 1.7g, Total Fat: 8.1g, Saturated Fat: 1.2g, Unsaturated Fat: 6.9g, Potassium: 529.1mg, Protein: 30.1g, Sodium: 232.7mg, Dietary Exchanges: 1 1/4 Fat, 1 Starch, 1 1/4 Vegetable, 3 1/2 Very Lean Meat.

NOTES

NOTES

Chapter 10

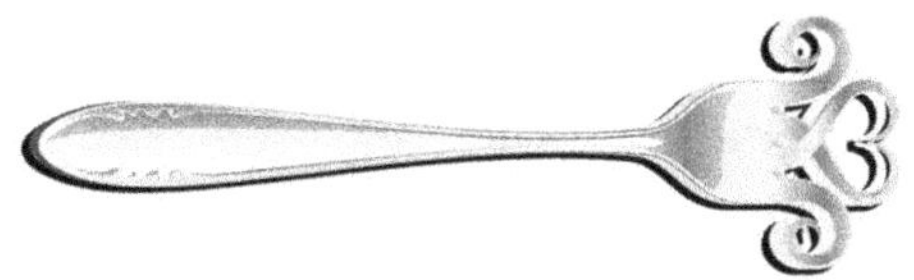

~DIABETIC SOUPS~

BROCCOLI AND POTATO SOUP

4 cups fresh broccoli, chopped
1 small onion, chopped
4 cups low-fat, unsalted chicken broth
1 cup evaporated non-fat skim milk
1 cup prepared instant mashed potatoes
salt and pepper to taste
1/4 cup low-fat shredded cheddar or American cheese

Combine broccoli, onion, and broth in large saucepan and bring to a boil. Reduce heat and cover. Reduce heat and simmer for about 10 minutes. Stir in milk. Slowly stir in prepared mashed potatoes. Cook and stir until bubbly and thickened. Season with salt and pepper. If it's too thick, stir in a little more milk or water. Ladle into soup bowls. Sprinkle about 1 Tbsp. of shredded cheese on top and serve. Makes 4 servings.

Calories: 216.2, Total Carbs: 26.1g, Dietary Fiber: 3.7g, Sugars: 11.3g, Total Fat: 3.9g, Saturated Fat: 1.8g, Unsaturated: 2.1g, Potassium: 548.7mg, Protein: 19.6g, Sodium: 432.8mg, Dietary Exchanges: 1/2 Milk, 1/2 Starch, 1 1/2 Vegetable.

BEEF, BARLEY, AND VEGETABLE SOUP

1 1/2 lbs. beef stew meat, trimmed and cubed
2 Tbsp. extra virgin olive oil
1 cup fresh chopped onion
2/3 cup fresh chopped celery
1/2 cup chopped carrots
1 clove garlic, minced
1 Tbsp. all-purpose flour
1 quart cold water
2 cups fat-free unsalted beef broth
1/2 tsp. ground marjoram leaves
1/2 tsp. ground thyme
1 bay leaf
1 can (14.5oz) diced tomatoes, do not drain
1 cup cut frozen green beans
1 cup fresh sliced parsnip
1/2 cup frozen sweet green peas
1/3 cup dry pearled barley
pinch salt and pepper

Heat oil over medium heat in a large pot and add the beef. Cook until brown on all sides, about 10 minutes. Stir in onion, celery, and garlic and cook for 5 minutes. Stir in flour and cook for 1 minute. Add water, broth, marjoram, thyme, and bay leaf and bring to a boil. Reduce heat, cover and simmer until beef is tender, about 1 hour to 1 1/2 hours. Raise the heat and add tomatoes, green beans, parsnips, peas, and barley. Bring to a boil. Reduce heat and simmer until veggies are tender and barley is cooked through, about 10 minutes. Add some salt and pepper to taste. Makes 8 servings.

Calories: 267, Total Carbs: 17.4g, Dietary Fiber: 4.1g, Sugars: 4.2g, Total Fat: 12.3g, Saturated Fat: 3.7g, Unsaturated Fat: 8.6g, Potassium: 455.7mg, Protein: 20.2g, Sodium: 156.5mg, Dietary Exchanges: 1 Fat, 2 1/2 Meat, 1/2 Starch, 1 1/2 Vegetable.

CHICKEN GUMBO

1/3 cup chopped onion
2 Tbsp. all-purpose flour
1 cup low sodium chicken broth
1/4 tsp. hot pepper sauce
1 can (14.5oz) stewed tomatoes
10oz. frozen sliced okra
3/4 lb. boneless, skinless chicken breasts
1/4 cup cold water
2 Tbsp. olive oil
1 Tbsp. chopped garlic
3 Tbsp. chopped celery
1/3 of a red pepper, chopped
1 tsp. Creole seasoning (or to taste)

Wash and pat dry the chicken breast and cut into 1-inch pieces. In a non-stick pot, heat olive oil over medium heat. Add chicken and cook for 5 minutes or until the chicken is done. Add garlic, onions, celery, and red bell pepper. Cook 5 minutes until veggies are crisp-tender. In a small cup, mix flour with 1/4 cup water and stir until smooth. Add the flour/water mixture, hot sauce, broth, tomatoes, and Creole seasoning to the pot. Cook for 3 minutes, stirring frequently. Add the okra, cover and simmer for about 8-10 minutes. Makes 6 servings.

Calories: 125.8, Total Carbs: 10.9g, Dietary Fiber: 2.1g, Sugars: 5.3g, Total Fat: 1.6g, Saturated Fat: 0.3g, Unsaturated Fat: 1.3g, Potassium: 513.6mg, Protein: 17.3g, Sodium: 366.1mg, Dietary Exchanges: 1 1/2 Meat, 1 1/2 Vegetable, 2 Very Lean Meat

Sharon Fox

OLD FASHIONED SOUP

1 1/2 lbs. pork shoulder, trimmed and cut into 1-inch cubes
2 Tbsp. vegetable oil
1 cup sliced carrots
2 stalks celery, cut into 1-inch pieces
2 potatoes, thinly sliced
1 packet Lipton onion soup mix
2 Tbsp. sugar
salt and pepper to taste
4 cups boiling water
2 beef bouillon cubes
28 oz. canned chopped tomatoes, in juice (unsalted)
1/4 tsp. oregano
dash of hot sauce (to taste)
10 oz. pkg. frozen okra, sliced

In Dutch oven, brown the meat in hot oil over medium-high heat. Add carrots, celery, potatoes, soup mix, sugar, salt, pepper, hot water, and bouillon cubes. Stir to mix well. Bring to a boil then lower heat to simmer. Cover and simmer 10 minutes. Stir in tomatoes, oregano, and a dash of hot sauce. Heat to boiling, reduce heat then cover and cook 45 minutes. Gently stir in okra during the last 15 minutes of cooking time. Makes 8 servings.

Calories: 269.2, Total Carbs: 20.8g, Dietary Fiber: 3.2g, Sugars: 8g, Total Fat: 10.6g, Saturated Fat: 3g, Unsaturated Fat: 7.6g, Potassium: 684.5mg, Protein: 21.8g, Sodium: 674.3mg, Dietary Exchanges: 1 Fat, 2 1/2 Meat, 1/2 Starch, 1 1/2 Vegetable

CRAB CHOWDER

1 Tbsp. canola oil
1 medium onion, chopped
3 medium stalks celery, thinly sliced
1 1/2 cups frozen sweet corn kernels, thawed
1 tsp. thyme
1/2 tsp. salt
1/4 tsp. pepper
2 cups low-sodium vegetable broth
1 cup fat-free evaporated milk
1 bay leaf
1 medium size potato, peeled and grated
3/4 lb. crab meat, cooked
1/4 cup fresh cilantro
dash of hot sauce (optional)

Heat oil in a large saucepan over medium heat. Add celery and onion and cook for 3 minutes. Stir in thyme, corn, salt, and pepper. Stir and cook for about 30 seconds. Add broth, evaporated milk, and bay leaf. Simmer for about 5 minutes. Grate the potato and add it to the chowder. Simmer for 5 minutes. Stir in crab meat and cilantro. Cook for 1 minute before serving. Makes 6 servings.

Calories: 216.3, Total Carbs: 20.8g, Dietary Fiber: 2.2g, Sugars: 6.3g, Total Fat: 6g, Saturated Fat: 2.1g, Unsaturated Fat: 3.9g, Potassium: 360.4mg, Protein: 18.5g, Sodium: 531.7mg, Dietary Exchanges: 1/2 Fat, 1/4 Milk, 1 Starch, 1/2 Vegetable, 2 Very Lean Meat.

VELVETY ASPARAGUS SOUP

1 Tbsp. unsalted butter
1 small onion, chopped
1 1/2 lbs. fresh asparagus, trimmed and chopped
1 can (14.5oz) fat-free reduced sodium chicken broth
1/2 tsp. salt
1/8 tsp. black pepper
1 cup cold water
1/4 cup heavy whipping cream

Melt butter in a large pot over medium heat and add the onions. Cook and stir until tender and slightly browned, about 8 minutes. Add the asparagus and cook about 5 minutes longer, stirring occasionally. Stir in the broth, salt, pepper, and water. Bring it to a boil over high heat, then lower heat, cover and simmer about 8 to 10 minutes until asparagus is tender. Remove pot from heat. Pour in blender in batches, leaving the center part of the cover out so steam can escape. Blend until smooth. Pour the blended mixture back into the pot, repeat until all of the asparagus mixture is blended. Once all of the blended asparagus mixture is all back in the pot, stir in the heavy cream and heat thoroughly. Do NOT allow it to boil or it will curdle. Just heat to a slow simmer until hot enough to enjoy. Serve immediately. Makes 4 servings.
For added flavor, top with some sliced green onions.

Calories: 130.9, Total Carbs: 10.9g, Dietary Fiber: 5g, Sugars: 4.9g, Total Fat: 8.4g, Saturated Fat: 5.2g, Unsaturated Fat: 3.2g, Potassium: 497mg, Protein: 6g, Sodium: 528.9mg, Dietary Exchanges: 2 Fat, 2 Vegetable.

BUTTERNUT SQUASH-SWEET POTATO SOUP

3 sweet potatoes, peeled and cubed
1 butternut squash, about 1 lb.
4 carrots, washed and peeled
1 stalk of celery
1 tsp. fresh ginger, minced
1/4 tsp. salt
1/4 tsp. fresh cracked black pepper
1 1/2 cups 2% milk

Cut the squash in half lengthwise and remove the seeds. Microwave, with the cut side down, in a dish with water about 1/2 inch deep for 15 minutes or until squash is soft. Meanwhile, steam the vegetables for about 15-20 minutes, until they are soft. Reserve cooking liquid in case you need to add some to your soup. Cool all vegetables until easy to handle.
Blend all of your vegetables in a blender or food processor, in batches if necessary. Add some of the cooking liquid if you need it to blend veggies. Return the blended mixture to the pot and add the milk, salt, pepper, and ginger. Heat and serve. Makes 8 servings.

Calories: 120, Total Carbs: 22g, Sugars: 2.5g,Total Fat: 1.4g, Saturated Fat: 1g Unsaturated Fat: 0.4g Protein, Dietary Fiber: 4g, Sodium: 310mg, Potassium: 789mg, Dietary Exchanges: 1 Starch, 1/2 Vegetable.

FRENCH ONION SOUP

cooking spray
1 1/2 lbs. yellow onions, thinly sliced
2 garlic cloves, minced
1 tsp. Stevia or Splenda
6 cups low-sodium vegetable broth
2 bay leaves
pinch of salt and pepper to taste
8 small slices bakery fresh French bread
4 oz. low sodium shredded Swiss cheese

Heat a Dutch oven or large pot coated with cooking spray over medium heat. Saute the onions and garlic, covered, over medium low heat for 8-10 minutes or until soft. Mix in the sugar substitute and cook until onions are golden brown. Add broth, water, and bay leaves and bring to a boil. Lower heat, cover with lid and simmer for 30 minutes. Take out the bay leaves, sprinkle with salt and pepper. Top each slice of bread with 1 Tbsp. of cheese. Broil in oven until cheese is melted. To serve, pour soup into bowls and top each with a toasted cheese bread! Makes 8 servings.

Calories: 115.1, Total Carbs: 12.1g, Dietary Fiber: 2g, Sugars: 4.9g, Total Fat:: 4.5g, Saturated Fat: 2.8g, Unsaturated Fat: 1.7g, Potassium: 153.6mg, Protein: 5.4g, Sodium: 110.9mg, Dietary Exchanges: 1/2 Fat, 1/2 Meat, 1 1/2 Vegetable

CHICKEN, KALE, AND LENTIL SOUP

1 Tbsp. olive oil
1 cup chopped onion
1 cup chopped carrots
2 cloves garlic, minced
6 cups low-sodium chicken broth
2 cups cold water
1 Tbsp. fresh basil, chopped
1 tsp. dried basil
4 cups kale, chopped
1/2 tsp. salt
1/8 tsp. black pepper
1 1/2 cups cooked chicken, cubed
1 tomato, seeded and chopped
1/2 cup cooked lentils, rinsed and drained

In a large saucepan, heat olive oil over medium heat. Add the onions, carrots, and garlic. Cook, covered, for about 6 minutes until the veggies are nearly tender. Stir occasionally. Add the chicken broth and water. Stir in the dried basil. Bring to a boil then reduce heat to simmer. Cover and simmer for 10 minutes. Stir in kale, salt, and pepper. Return to boil, reduce to simmer and cook covered for 10 more minutes. Stir in the chicken, tomato, fresh basil, and lentils. Cover and simmer for about 8 more minutes until kale and lentils are tender. Makes 6 servings.

Calories: 160, Total Carbs: 14.4g, Dietary Fiber: 3.5g, Sugars: 3.5g, Total Fat: 4.4g, Saturated Fat: 0.8g, Unsaturated Fat: 3.6g, Potassium: 631.9mg, Protein: 16.4g, Sodium: 611.8mg, Dietary Exchanges: 1/2 Fat, 2 Vegetable, 1 1/2 Very Lean Meat

SMOKED TURKEY AND LIMA BEAN SOUP

1 Tbsp. olive oil
1 yellow onion, sliced thin
3 cloves garlic, chopped
1/2 tsp. ground thyme
3 cups reduced sodium, fat-free chicken broth
1 carrot, diced
3 cups frozen lima beans, thawed
1/2 lb smoked lemon pepper deli turkey breast, diced
1 Tbsp. chopped green onion

Heat oil in a large pot over medium high heat and add onion. Saute until soft, about 3 minutes. Add the garlic and thyme. cook for an additional minute, careful not to brown. Add the broth and carrots and bring to a boil. Stir in beans and turkey. Lower heat, cover, and simmer about 5 minutes. If soup gets too thick, just add a little hot water or extra broth. Serve topped with green onions. Makes 8 servings.

Calories: 114, Total Carbs: 16.1g, Dietary Fiber: 3.5g, Sugars: 1g, Total Fat: 2g, Saturated Fat: 0.3g, Unsaturated Fat: 1.7g, Potassium: 355.7mg, Protein: 6.8g, Sodium: 270.5 mg, Dietary Exchanges: 1/4 Fat, 1 Starch, 1/2 Vegetable.

PEACH SOUP

1 1/2 lbs. fresh peaches sliced, or 28oz. can sliced peaches, drained
2 cups plain non-fat plain yogurt
1 cup orange juice
1 cup pineapple juice
1 Tbsp. fresh lemon juice
2 Tbsp. sugar
1 Tbsp. almond extract

Puree the peaches in a food processor until smooth. Add the yogurt, orange juice, pineapple juice, lemon juice, sugar, and almond extract. Blend until smooth. Chill until ready to serve. Makes a lovely, cool soup for hot summer days or serve as an elegant course when you want to serve a special meal. Makes 10 servings.

Calories: 85.6, Total Carbs: 17.9g, Dietary Fiber: 1g, Sugars: 16.7g, Total Fat: 0.3g, Saturated Fat: 0g, Unsaturated Fat: 0.3g, Potassium: 177.3mg, Protein 3.2g, Sodium: 61.5mg, Dietary Exchanges: 1 Fruit, 1/4 Milk

SEAFOOD WONTON SOUP

2 oz. large raw shrimp
2 oz. large scallops
3 oz. fresh cod fillets, chopped
1 Tbsp. chives, finely chopped
1 tsp. cooking sherry
1 egg white
1/2 tsp. sesame oil
1/4 tsp. salt
pinch white pepper
20 wonton wrappers
2 leaves of romaine lettuce
3 3/4 cups fish stock
pinch of fresh cilantro
fresh chives for garnish

Peel and devein the shrimp. Rinse and dry them and chop into small pieces. Rinse and dry the scallops, chop into same size pieces as the shrimp. Put the cod in a food processor and process until a paste is formed. Scrape the paste into a bowl and stir in the shrimp, scallops, chives, sherry, sesame oil, salt and pepper. Lightly beat egg white and add to the seafood filling. Mix well, cover, and chill for 20 minutes.
Place 1 tsp. of the mixture in the center of each wonton wrapper. Bring corners together to meet at the top and twist together to enclose the filling. If you want to be fancy, tie the tops with a fresh chive. Boil a large pot of water and drop wontons in, one at a time. When the water returns to a boil, lower the heat and simmer gently for 5 minutes or until wontons float to the surface. Drain and divide them among 4 heated bowls. Add a leaf of lettuce to each bowl. Bring the fish stock to a boil. Ladle it on top of the lettuce and garnish each bowl with cilantro leaves and chives. Makes 4 servings.

Calories: 177.8, Total Carbs: 16.2g, Dietary Fiber: 0.6g, Sugars: 0.8g, Total Fat: 3.1g, Saturated Fat: 0.6g, Unsaturated Fat: 2.5g, Potassium: 766.5mg, Protein: 19.2g, Sodium: 594mg, Dietary Exchanges: 1 Starch, 1 1/4 Very Lean Meat

KICKED UP BEEF STEW

1 1/2 lb. boneless beef chuck roast
1 lb. fresh butternut squash, cubed
2 small onions, cut into wedges
2 cloves garlic, minced
14oz. beef broth
8oz. salt-free tomato sauce
2 Tbsp. Worcestershire sauce
1 tsp. dry mustard
1/4 tsp. black pepper
1/8 tsp. ground allspice
4 tsp. cornstarch
2 Tbsp. cold water
9oz. frozen Italian cut green beans

Remove all excess fat from meat and cut into 1-inch pieces. Place into a 3 1/2 to 4 quart slow cooker. Add cubed squash, onions, and garlic. Now add the beef broth, tomato sauce, Worcestershire sauce, dry mustard, pepper, and allspice. Stir to blend. Cover and cook on low setting for 8 to 10 hours (or on high 4 to 5 hours). During last 15 minutes, combine the 2 Tbsp. cold water with 4 tsp. cornstarch and add it to the slow cooker. Stir and finish cooking for 15 minutes or until gravy has thickened. Makes 6 servings.

Calories: 333.7, Total Carbs: 28.4g, Dietary Fiber: 5g, Sugars: 7.8g, Total Fat: 9.8g, Saturated Fat: 3.5g, Unsaturated Fat: 6.3g, Potassium: 1,219.3mg, Protein: 31.2g, Sodium: 454.6mg, Sodium: 454.6mg, Dietary Exchanges: 3 1/2 Meat, 4 1/2 Vegetable

Sharon Fox

THAI OMLET SOUP

1 egg
1 Tbsp. peanut oil
3 3/4 cups low-sodium vegetable broth
2 carrots, finely diced
4 cups Savoy cabbage, shredded
2 Tbsp. low-sodium soy sauce
1/2 tsp. sugar
1/2 tsp. black pepper
1 sprig parsley or cilantro for garnish

Crack egg into a small bowl and beat lightly with a fork. In a small non-stick frying pan, heat the oil over medium heat and add egg to the pan, swirling around to coat the pan. Cook until the underside is golden brown. Slide the egg out of pan and roll up into a log. Slice into 1/4- inch rounds and set aside for garnish. In a large pan, combine the vegetable broth, carrots, and cabbage. Bring to a boil, reduce heat and simmer 5 minutes. Add soy sauce, sugar, and pepper. Stir well and pour into warmed bowls. Lay the egg rounds on surface of each portion, garnish with cilantro or parsley leaves. Makes 4 servings.

* If you can't find Savoy cabbage, Bok Choy may be used.

Calories: 105.3, Total Carbs: 11.2g, Dietary Fiber: 3.6g, Sugars: 4.4g, Total Fat: 4.9g, Saturated Fat: 1g, Unsaturated Fat: 3.9g, Potassium: 298.7mg, Protein: 3.8g, Sodium: 384.7mg, Dietary Exchanges: 1 Fat, 1 1/4 Vegetable

NOTES

NOTES

Chapter 11

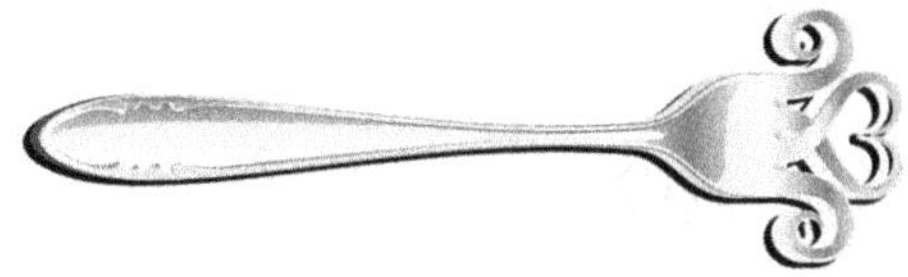

~DIABETIC DESSERTS~

LIGHT ALMOND COOKIES

3 egg whites
1/8 tsp. salt
1 cup sugar
1 tsp. vanilla extract
1/2 cup whole almonds, toasted and finely chopped
cooking spray

Spray two cookie sheets with cooking spray. preheat the oven to 250 degrees. Beat the egg whites with electric mixer until soft peaks are formed. Add the salt, now slowly add in the sugar as mixture is beating. Add vanilla. Continue to beat until mixture forms stiff peaks but not dry. Gently fold in the almonds. Drop by teaspoonfuls onto sheet, lifting spoon from the center of each one to make a little peak on top of each cookie. You'll need to work quickly so the batter does not spread. Bake for about 25 minutes, until the cookies are light brown and hard to the touch on top. Carefully remove from cookie sheets and place on a wire rack to cool. Makes 40 cookies. 1 cookie per serving.

Calories: 16, Total Carbs: 3.7g, Dietary Fiber: 0.1g, Sugars: 3.6g, Total Fat: 0.2g, Saturated Fat: 0g, Unsaturated Fat: 0.2g, Potassium: 7.3mg, Protein: 0.4g, Sodium: 11.4mg, Dietary Exchanges: Other Carbohydrate: 0.2g, Starch: 0g, Very Lean Meat: 0

BUTTERSCOTCH-APPLE DESSERT SQUARES

3 large apples, grated
1/2 cup margarine, softened (80% fat)
3/4 cup brown sugar
2 eggs
1/2 cup vanilla non-fat yogurt
1/2 cup 2% milk
1 tsp. vanilla extract
1 1/2 cups all purpose flour
1/2 cup whole wheat flour
1 tsp. baking soda
pinch of salt
1 cup butterscotch baking chips

Cream together the margarine and sugar. Blend in the eggs, yogurt, milk, and vanilla. Sift the dry ingredients together and blend into the creamed mixture. Stir in the grated apples and butterscotch chips. Spread the batter into a 9-inch square baking pan which has been coated with a butter-flavored vegetable cooking spray. Bake at 350 degrees for about 45 minutes, until lightly browned. Cool completely and cut into 25 squares (5 squares x 5 squares). Serving size is one square.

Calories: 166.4, Total Carbs: 23.7g, Dietary Fiber: 1.1g, Sugars: 15.2g, Total Fat: 6.7g, Saturated Fat: 2.9g, Unsaturated Fat: 3.8g, Potassium: 75.9mg, Protein: 2.1g, Sodium: 107.3mg, Dietary Exchanges: 1 1/4 Fat, 1 Other Carbohydrate, 1/2 Starch.

SIMPLE BAKED CUSTARD

2 eggs
2 cups fat-free milk
1/3 cup liquid brown sugar
2 tsp. vanilla extract

In a small bowl, lightly beat the eggs. Add all remaining ingredients and beat well to combine. Pour this mixture into five 6oz. ramekins or custard cups. Place the filled cups in a baking pan. Fill the baking pan to 1-inch with hot water. Bake for 45 minutes at 350 degrees, until a knife inserted in the center comes out clean. Cover with plastic wrap and chill until serving time. Serve with fresh berries! Makes 5 servings.

* When you cover with plastic wrap, allow the plastic to lay directly on the custard to prevent a skin from forming.

Calories: 127.9, Total Carbs: 20.7g, Dietary Fiber: 0g, Sugars: 20g, Total Fat: 2g, Saturated Fat: 0.6g, Unsaturated Fat: 1.4g, Potassium: 83mg, Protein: 6.1g, Sodium: 86.2mg, Dietary Exchanges: 1/4 Meat, 1/2 Milk, 1 Other Carbohydrate.

BANANA CREAM

1 large banana
4 Tbsp. Cool Whip Lite
1 cup plain non-fat Greek yogurt
1 tsp. vanilla or rum extract
4 graham crackers, crushed
3 strawberries sliced OR 6 slices of banana

Place the large banana2 Tbsp. of the Cool Whip, yogurt, and vanilla extract in a blender and puree until smooth. Divide the crushed graham crackers between 3 serving glasses or bowls. Place 2/3 cup portions of the puree into each dish. Top with remaining Cool Whip. Add the strawberries or banana slices and serve immediately. Makes 3 servings.

Calories: 123.3, Total Carbs: 22.8g, Dietary Fiber: 1.5g, Sugars: 13.8g, Total Fat: 1.5g, Saturated Fat: 0.9g, Unsaturated Fat: 0.6g, Potassium: 182.8mg, Protein: 4.9g, Sodium: 87.4mg, Dietary Exchanges: 1 Fruit, 1/2 Milk.

BETTER THAN BANANA SPLIT DESSERT

6 1/2 honey graham crackers (two 1 1/2 squares per sheet)
1 small box sugar-free, fat-free instant vanilla pudding mix
2 cups fat-free milk
8 oz. light cream cheese, softened
10 oz. unsweetened crushed pineapple, drained
4 bananas, sliced
8 oz. Cool Whip Lite
3 Tbsp. chopped pecans

Cover the bottom of a 9x13-inch pan with graham crackers. In a medium size bowl, make the pudding with 2 cups fat-free milk, according to package directions. Add the softened cream cheese to the pudding and mix well. Spread over the graham crackers in the pan. Spread the crushed pineapple over the pudding mixture. Top with sliced bananas then add Cool Whip. Sprinkle the pecans on top. Makes 16 servings.

Calories: 143.7, Total Carbs: 22.1g, Dietary Fiber: 1.5g,Sugars: 11.8g, Total Fat: 5.1g, Saturated Fat: 3g, Unsaturated Fat: 2.1g, Potassium: 29.6mg, Protein: 3.2g, Sodium: 179.4mg, Dietary Exchanges: 1/2 Fat, 1/2 Fruit, 1/4 Starch.

BLACK AND WHITE CHEESECAKE BARS

12 oz. (1 1/2 blocks) fat-free cream cheese, softened
2 1/4 cups sugar
1 cup liquid egg substitute
1 Tbsp. vanilla extract
1 cup stone ground whole wheat pastry flour
1/2 cup semi-sweet chocolate chips, melted
3 Tbsp. unsweetened cocoa powder
1/3 cup chopped walnuts (optional)

Preheat oven to 325 degrees. Spray an 8x8-inch baking dish with cooking spray and set aside. In a large bowl, beat the cream cheese until smooth. Add the sugar and beat well. Add egg substitute and vanilla. Beat until sugar is dissolved. Slowly beat in the flour and mix well. Remove 1 1/2 cups of the batter into a separate small bowl. Stir the melted chocolate and cocoa into the remaining batter. Mix well and pour into the prepared baking dish. Drop the white batter over the chocolate batter by spoonfuls and top with nuts, if using. Use a knife to swirl slightly. Bake about 55 minutes until lightly browned. Cool completely and then cover and chill. Cut into 16 bars before serving. Makes 16 servings.

Calories: 160, Total Carbs: 32g, Dietary Fiber: 1.5g, Sugars: 20.2g, Total Fat: 3.9g, Saturated Fat: 1.5g, Unsaturated Fat: 2.4g, Potassium: 26.8mg, Protein: 2.7g, Sodium: 33.9mg, Dietary Exchanges: 1 Fat, 1 1/4 Other Carbohydrate, 1/4 Starch

APPLE-SCOTCH PUDDING DESSERT

1 small. package (4-serving size) sugar-free butterscotch pudding mix
1/3 cup non-fat dry milk powder
1/2 tsp. apple pie spice
1 1/2 cups cold water
1/2 cup unsweetened applesauce
2 oz. seedless raisins
1/4 cup whipped cream topping

In a medium size bowl, combine the dry pudding mix, dry milk powder, and apple pie spice. Add the water, applesauce, and raisins. Using a wire whisk, mix all ingredients until completely combined and smooth. Pour into 4 dessert dishes and chill for 30 minutes. Right before serving, top with whipped cream topping. Makes 4 servings.

Calories: 57.1, Total Carbs: 10.6g, Dietary Fiber: 0.3g, Sugars: 6.9g, Total Fat: 0.8g, Saturated Fat: 0.5g, Unsaturated Fat: 0.3g, Potassium: 93.5mg, Protein: 2.3g, Sodium: 82.8mg, Dietary Exchanges: 1/4 Fruit.

Sharon Fox

BLUEBERRY-LEMON TART

35 fat-free Vanilla Wafers cookies, crushed (1 1/2 cups)
1 egg white, beaten
1 Tbsp. butter, melted
1 1/4 cups fat-free milk
1 (3oz) pkg. lemon instant pudding mix
1 1/2 tsp. fresh lemon zest
1 cup Cool Whip (low-fat), thawed

Blueberry Topping:
2 Tbsp. sugar
1 tsp. cornstarch
3 Tbsp. cold water
1 1/2 cups blueberries (fresh or frozen)
1 Tbsp. fresh lemon juice

Heat oven to 400 degrees. Spray a 9x1-inch tart pan (with removable bottom) lightly with cooking spray. Mix the crushed cookies, egg white, and butter until crumbly. Press into the bottom and up the sides of tart pan. Bake 8-10 minutes until light golden brown in color. Cool completely.

In a medium size bowl, beat the pudding mix, milk, and lemon zest with an electric mixer on low speed until smooth- about 2 minutes. Chill for about 5 minutes. Fold in the whipped topping and spread into the cooled crust. Cover and chill at least 2 hours. Serve with blueberry topping.

For the topping: Mix the sugar, cornstarch, and water in a 1-quart saucepan. Stir in 1/2 cup of the blueberries. Heat to boiling then reduce heat to medium low setting. Cook 5 minutes or until mixture is slightly thickened. Stir in lemon juice and remove from heat. Cool 10 minutes. Stir in the remaining blueberries. Cover and chill at least 1 hour.

This entire recipe makes 12 servings.

Calories: 118.6, Total Carbs: 23.9g, Dietary Fiber: 0.5g, Sugars: 13.3g, Total Fat:1.9g, Saturated Fat: 1.3g, Unsaturated Fat: 0.6g, Potassium: 13.4mg, Protein: 2.3g, Sodium: 109.3mg, Dietary Exchanges: 1 Other Carbohydrate.

ORANGE CAKE

1/3 cup margarine (80% fat), melted
1/4 cup granulated brown sugar substitute
1/4 cup Stevia or Sweet-n-Low
1 egg
1 1/4 cups all purpose flour
2 tsp. low-sodium baking powder
1/2 tsp. baking soda
1/4 tsp. cinnamon
1/3 cup seedless raisins
2/3 cup frozen orange juice concentrate, thawed
cooking spray

Preheat your oven to 350 degrees. Combine the margarine, sugars, and egg. Beat on high speed for 2 minutes with an electric mixer. In a separate bowl, combine the flour, baking soda, baking powder, and cinnamon. Stir in the raisins. Alternately add the flour mixture with the orange juice, beginning and ending with the flour mixture. Beat well after each addition to mix well. Spoon the batter into an 8-inch baking pan that has been coated with cooking spray. Bake for 25-30 minutes. Cool completely and then cut into 9 squares. Makes 9 servings.

Calories: 184.4, Total Carbs: 27.3g, Dietary Fiber: 1g, Sugars: 12.2g, Total Fat: 7.5g, Saturated Fat: 1.5g, Unsaturated Fat: 6g, Potassium: 1,036.8mg, Protein: 3.2g, Sodium" 158.8mg, Dietary Exchanges: 1 1/4 Fat, 1 Fruit, 1 Starch

DELICIOUS DIABETIC APPLE-CINNAMON CHEESECAKE

16 oz. fat-free cream cheese
1 pkg. (4 serving pkg.) sugar-free instant vanilla pudding mix
2/3 cup non-fat dry skim milk
1 cup unsweetened apple juice
1 tsp. cinnamon
1/4 cup fat-free whipped topping
1/2 cup seedless raisins
1 graham cracker crust
3 Tbsp. apple butter

Beat softened cream cheese in a mixing bowl until smooth and creamy. Whisk in the dry pudding mix, dry milk powder, and apple juice using a wire whisk. Blend in the cinnamon, whipped topping, and raisins. Spread into pie crust and chill for at least 30 minutes before cutting. Cut into 8 servings. Top each slice with 1 tsp. apple butter. Makes 8 servings.

Calories: 181.4, Total Carbs: 25.3g, Dietary Fiber: 0.3g, Sugars: 14.9g, Total Fat: 6.2g, Saturated Fat: 1.3g, Unsaturated Fat: 4.9g, Potassium: 171.8mg, Protein: 5.4g, Sodium: 211.6mg, Dietary Exchanges: 1 Fat, 1 Other Carbohydrate.

FRESH CHERRY-OATMEAL COOKIES

olive oil cooking spray
1/4 cup brown sugar
1/4 cup honey
1/2 cup margarine, softened
2 eggs
1/2 tsp. baking soda
1 1/2 tsp. vanilla extract
1 cup unbleached, all purpose flour
2 cups old fashioned rolled oats
1 cup fresh cherries, pitted and chopped (20 cherries)
1/2 cup chopped walnuts
2 cups bran flakes cereal, crushed

Preheat oven to 350 degrees. Lightly spray 2 cookie sheets with olive oil cooking spray. Beat the sugar, honey, margarine, eggs, baking soda, and vanilla extract in a large mixing bowl on medium speed for about 2 minutes. Stir in the oats, flour, chopped cherries, walnuts, and bran flakes. Chill for 15 minutes. Drop spoonfuls of the cookie mixture onto the cookie sheets about 2 inches apart. Bake about 12-15 minutes or until lightly browned. Cool for 3-4 minutes on the tray and then remove cookies to a wire rack to finish cooling. Makes about 42 cookies, 1 per serving.
*You may substitute other fresh fruit in place of cherries if you want.

Calories: 69, Total Carbs: 8.1g, Dietary Fiber: 0.9g, Sugars: 2.1g, Total Fat: 3.5g, Saturated Fat: 0.5g, Unsaturated Fat: 3g, Potassium: 19mg, Protein: 1.7g, Sodium: 52mg, Dietary Exchanges: 1/2 Fat: 1/2 Starch.

YUMMY CHOCOLATE RICE KRISPIES TREATS

2 Tbsp. unsalted butter
1 oz. unsweetened baking chocolate, finely chopped
7oz. jar marshmallow cream
2 Tbsp. unsweetened cocoa powder
1 tsp. vanilla extract
6 cups. Rice Krispies cereal

Spray a 9x13-inch baking pan with cooking spray and set aside. In a large pot melt butter and chocolate over low heat. Stir in the marshmallow cream, cocoa, and vanilla until smooth. Remove from heat and stir in the cereal, coating well with the hot mixture. Spread into the baking pan. Lightly spray your hands with cooking spray and press the mixture evenly in the pan. Let cool completely and then cut into 24 squares. Makes 24 servings.

Calories: 65.8, Total Carbs: 11.9g, Dietary Fiber: 0.2g, Sugars: 4.4g, Total Fat: 1.6g, Saturated Fat: 1g, Unsaturated Fat: 0.6g, Potassium: 15.1mg, Protein: 0.7g, Sodium: 57.6mg, Dietary Exchanges: 1/4 Fat, 1/2 Other Carbohydrate, 1/4 Starch.

CHOCOLATE CAKE

3/4 cup margarine, at room temperature
1/4 cup sugar
1/2 cup liquid egg substitute, at room temp.
1/3 cup unsweetened cocoa powder
1/3 cup granulated sugar substitute
2 tsp. vanilla extract
2 cups white cake flour
2 tsp. low sodium baking powder
1/4 cup non-fat dry milk
1 cup water, room temp.

Grease a 9-inch square baking pan and set aside. Preheat your oven to 350 degrees. Cream the margarine and sugar together until fluffy. Beat in the egg substitute, sugar substitute, and vanilla until sugar is dissolved. In a separate bowl, mix the flour, baking powder, dry milk, and cocoa powder. Add the dry mixture alternately with 1 cup of water to the creamed mixture. Mix until smooth and then spread into the prepared baking pan. Bake for 30-35 minutes and cool completely. Makes 16 servings.

Calories: 143, Total Carbs: 15.3g, Dietary Fiber: 0.8g, Sugars: 3.1g, Total Fat: 8.5g, Saturated Fat: 1.6g, Unsaturated Fat: 6.9g, Potassium: 124.6mg, Protein: 1.9g, Sodium: 85.9mg, Dietary Exchanges: 2 Fat, 1/2 Starch.

CHOCOLATE SAUCE

3 Tbsp. unsweetened cocoa powder
4 tsp. cornstarch
1/3 cup non-fat dry skim milk
1/8 tsp. salt
1 1/2 cups cold water
1 Tbsp. margarine
2 tsp. vanilla
10 packets of Equal, Stevia, or Splenda

In a small saucepan, mix the cocoa powder, cornstarch, dry milk, and salt. Stir in water until smooth. Add the margarine and cook over low heat, stirring occasionally. Bring this mixture to a boil and reduce to simmer for about 2 minutes, stirring constantly. Remove from heat and stir in vanilla and sweetener. Pour into a glass jar and refrigerate until ready to use. Makes 12 servings. (Each serving size is 2 Tbsp.)
Bring to room temperature before serving.

Calories: 24.2, Total Carbs: 2.6g, Dietary Fiber: 0.5g, Sugars: 1.1g, Total Fat: 1.1g, Saturated Fat: 0.3g, Unsaturated Fat: 0.8g, Potassium: 55.7mg, Protein: 1g, Sodium: 45.9mg, Dietary Exchanges: 0.2 Fat, Milk 0.1, 0 Other Carbohydrate.

CHOCOLATE CHIP COOKIES

8 Tbsp. margarine, softened
1 cup packed light brown sugar
1/2 cup sugar
1 egg
1 tsp. vanilla extract
2 1/2 cup all purpose flour
1/2 tsp. baking soda
1/2 tsp. salt
1/3 cup fat-free milk
6 oz. semi-sweet chocolate chips

Preheat oven to 375 degrees. Using an electric mixer, beat margarine and sugars until fluffy. Beat in eggs and vanilla. Combine flour, baking soda, and salt. Gradually beat this dry mixture into the margarine mixture, alternately with milk, start and finish with the dry ingredients. Stir in the chocolate chips. Chill for 30 minutes to 1 hour. Spoon into rounds onto a greased cookie sheet. Bake for 10 minutes or until golden brown. Cool on wire racks. Makes 60 servings (1 cookie per serving).

Calories: 69.5, Total Carbs: 11.2g, Dietary Fiber: 0.1g, Sugars: 5.3g, Total Fat: 2.4g, Saturated Fat: 0.8g, Unsaturated Fat: 1.6g, Potassium: 6.8mg, Protein: 0.9g, Sodium: 46.9mg, Dietary Exchanges: 1/2 Fat, 1/2 Other Carbohydrate.

CREAMY RICE PUDDING

1 small box sugar-free instant vanilla pudding mix
3 1/2 cups fat-free milk
4 oz. low-fat whipped topping, thawed
1 tsp. almond extract
1 cup seedless raisins
2 cups medium grain white rice, cooked

In a medium size bowl, whisk together the dry pudding mix and milk for 2 minutes. Stir in the whipped topping, almond extract, raisins, and rice. Stir until well combined. Serve immediately or chill and serve cold. You may sprinkle a little nutmeg or cinnamon on top to garnish.
This is a wonderful way to get rid of leftover rice! Makes 14 servings

Calories: 61.2, Total Carbs: 11.4g, Dietary Fiber: 0.1g, Sugars: 3.3g, Total Fat: 0.2g, Saturated Fat: 0.1g, Unsaturated Fat: 0.1g, Potassium: 8.5 mg, Protein: 2.9g, Sodium: 38.2mg, Dietary Exchanges: 1/2 Fruit, 1/4 Milk, 1/2 Starch.

NO-CRUST FRUIT CUSTARD PIE

Butter flavored cooking spray
2 cups fresh or frozen sliced peaches, thawed (or pears or apples)
2 2/3 cups whole milk
1/3 cup all purpose flour
1/2 cup granulated Stevia or Splenda
1 1/2 tsp. vanilla extract
2 eggs
1/3 cup soy flour

Preheat your oven to 375 degrees. Coat the bottom of a 9-inch pie pan with cooking spray. Arrange the fruit of choice in bottom of pie plate.
In a mixing bowl, whisk together the milk, flour, soy flour, sweetener, vanilla, and eggs. Pour this custard mixture over the fruit. Bake 1 hour and 10 minutes or until a toothpick inserted in the center comes out clean. Cool and serve, or chill and serve later. Makes 8 servings.

Calories: 124.9, Total Carbs: 14.6g, Dietary Fiber: 1.1g, Sugars: 7.2g, Total Fat: 4.6g, Saturated Fat: 2.2g, Unsaturated Fat: 2.4g, Potassium: 84.8mg, Protein: 6g,Sodium: 57.2mg, Dietary Exchanges: 1/4 Milk, 1/4 Starch, 1/4 Very Lean Meat.

DEEP DISH APPLE PIE

6 cups fresh apples, peeled and thinly sliced
1/4 cup sugar
1 tsp. cinnamon
1 Tbsp. Argo corn starch
1/8 tsp. salt
1/2 cup all purpose flour
1/4 cup whole wheat flour
1 pinch ground nutmeg
3 Tbsp. butter or margarine
2 Tbsp. cold water
1 tsp. whole milk

Place apples in a 2 quart square baking dish. In a small bowl combine the sugar and cinnamon and set aside 1 tsp. of this mixture. Stir the cornstarch and salt into the remaining sugar mixture and sprinkle evenly over apples in baking dish. In a medium bowl stir together the flours and nutmeg. use a pastry blender to cut in the butter until crumbly. Sprinkle 1 Tbsp. of the water over the mixture and gently toss with a fork. Push the moistened dough to one side and repeat, using 1 Tbsp. of the water at a time until all dough is moistened. Form into a ball. Flatten dough on a lightly floured surface. Roll from center to edges into a 10-inch square. Cut a few decorative vents into the pastry. Carefully place the pastry over the apples. Use a fork to press edges to sides of dish. Brush the pastry with milk and sprinkle with reserved sugar and cinnamon mixture. Bake in a 375 degree oven for about 40 minutes or until apples are tender and crust is golden brown. Serve warm. Makes 8 servings.

Calories: 150.3, Total Carbs: 27.3g, Dietary Fiber: 2.8g, Sugars: 14.8g, Total Fat: 4.6g, Saturated Fat: 2.8g, Unsaturated Fat: 1.8g, Potassium: 113.9mg, Protein: 1.6g, Sodium: 68.2mg, Dietary Exchanges: 1 Fat, 1 Fruit, 1/4 Other Carbohydrate, 1/2 Starch.

QUICK APPLE-PEAR CRISP

1 1/2 medium apples, peeled, cored, and thinly sliced
1 1/2 medium pears, cored and sliced thin
1/2 cup quick cooking rolled oats
1/4 cup light brown sugar, packed
3 Tbsp. all purpose flour
1 tsp. cinnamon
1/4 tsp. nutmeg
4 tsp. cold margarine, diced

Spray a 9-inch square microwave-safe baking dish with cooking spray. Put all the apples and pears in the dish. Place in the microwave with a vented cover and cook on high for 3 minutes. Stir and cook for an additional 3 minutes. The fruit should be partially cooked and crisp-tender.
While the fruit is cooking, combine the oatmeal, sugar, flour, cinnamon, and nutmeg in a small bowl. Cut the cold margarine into the mixture with a pastry blender, fork, or two knives. The mixture should now look like coarse crumbs. Sprinkle this mixture over the partially cooked fruit and microwave until fruit is soft. This should take about 6 minutes. Makes 4 servings.
*You can add some fresh cranberries or blueberries for a special treat!

Calories: 218.3, Total Carbs: 43.3g, Dietary Fiber: 5g, Sugars: 26g, Total Fat: 5g, Saturated Fat: 0.8g, Unsaturated Fat: 4.2g, Potassium: 10.6mg, Protein: 2.6g, Sodium: 48.3mg, Dietary Exchanges: 1 Fat, 1 1/4 Fruit, 1 Other Carbohydrate, 1 Starch.

SWEET POTATO OR PUMPKIN HOLIDAY PIE

1 frozen 9-inch pie crust
2 cups solid pack canned pumpkin or baked sweet potato
12 oz. evaporated milk
3 eggs
3/4 cup granulated sweetener (Splenda or Stevia)
1 tsp. vanilla extract
1 tsp. cinnamon
1/4 tsp. ground ginger
1/4 tsp. ground nutmeg
1/4 tsp. salt
10 Tbsp. Cool Whip (fat-free)

Preheat oven to 400 degrees. In a medium size bowl, add the pumpkin or sweet potato, evaporated milk, and eggs. Beat with an electric mixer on medium speed until well combined. Add sweetener, vanilla, cinnamon, ginger, nutmeg, and salt. Mix well. Place the pie shell on a cookie sheet. Pour the filling into pie shell and bake for 35-40 minutes or until set. Cool on a wire rack. Serve at room temperature. Top with a Tbsp. of Cool Whip (fat-free), if desired. Makes 10 servings.

Calories: 137.1, Total Carbs: 16.1g (pumpkin) or 33.2g (sweet potato), Dietary Fiber: 2.1g, Sugars: 4.9g, Total Fat: 7.1g, Saturated Fat: 3.3g, Unsaturated Fat: 3.8g, Potassium: 118.8mg, Protein: 5.6g, Sodium: 173.4mg, Dietary Exchanges: 1/4 Fat, 1/4 Meat, 1/4 Milk, 1/2 Other Carbohydrate.

NOTES

Chapter 12

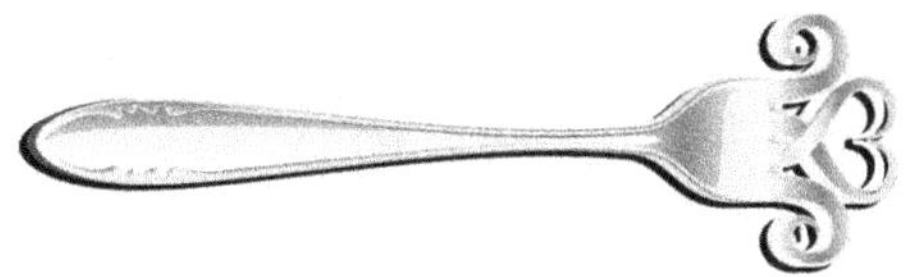

~VEGETARIAN LIFESTYLE~

Many people become vegetarian overnight. They totally give up meat, fish, and poultry instantly. Others make a gradual change. It all depends on what works best for you. There are different types of vegetarian.

Lacto-Ovo Vegetarians eat both dairy products and eggs. This is the most common vegetarian diet. Many will only eat free-range eggs because of the welfare objections to the intensive farming of hens.

Lacto Vegetarians eat dairy products, but avoid eggs.

Vegans do not eat any dairy products or any other products which come from an animal. They say, "If it has parents or a face, we don't eat it."

Some people are vegetarian for religious reasons. No matter what the case may be, we must realize that vegetarianism is growing more popular every year. Becoming a vegetarian can only be as easy or as hard as you choose to make it. Some people enjoy planning the elaborate meals, while others like quick and easy vegetarian dishes. In any instance, the main concern should be proper nutrition.

Any diet, including vegetarian, has its ups and downs. You may want to speak with your doctor, a dietician, or other nutritional expert before changing to any type of special diet. Remember that the main concern is always your health. If you already have health issues, you definitely want to check with your doctor as certain diets can be very dangerous for you.

Vegetarians and Nutrition

Protein

Vegetarians can easily meet their protein needs by eating a varied diet, as long as they consume enough calories to maintain their weight. A mixture of proteins throughout the day will provide enough essential amino acids. Great sources of protein are: beans, lentils, tofu, nuts, seeds, tempeh, and chickpeas. Other common foods can quickly add protein to your diet. These include: whole grain bread, greens, potatoes, and corn.

Iron

Sources of iron include: dried fruits, mushrooms, baked potatoes, dried beans, cashews, spinach, tofu, chard, bulgur, and several iron-fortified foods such as cereals, instant oatmeal, and veggie-meats. To increase the amount of iron absorbed in a meal, eat a food with lots of vitamin C, such as citrus fruits or juices, tomatoes, or broccoli. Using iron cookware will also add to your iron intake.

Calcium

Sources of calcium include: collard greens, broccoli, mustard greens, kale, low-fat dairy products, fortified soymilk, and fortified orange juice.

Vitamin B-12

The recommended intake for vitamin B-12 is very low for adults. This vitamin comes primarily from animal derived foods. A diet containing dairy products or eggs provides adequate vitamin B-12. Good non-animal sources would be: some cereals that are fortified with B-12, nutritional yeast, and soymilk. Contrary to popular belief, sea vegetables and tempeh are not reliable sources for B-12. To be on the safe side, if you aren't eating dairy products or fortified foods regularly, you should take a non-animal derived supplement.

Omega-3

To maximize production of omega-3 fatty acids that are made by your own body and found in fish, you should include good sources of alpha-linolenic acid in your diet. Great sources would be: flaxseed, flaxseed oil, canola oil, tofu, walnuts, and soybeans. You can also check your brand of soymilk, it should be fortified with DHA. Vitamin supplements containing microalgae-derived DHA would be good as well.

When changing over to a vegetarian diet, do your homework first. Experiment with several recipes and vegetarian products so that you can acquire the taste for the fresh change! A great way to start is by visiting your local whole food store, health food store, produce market, and look for some new healthy dishes in some restaurants. You'd be surprised at the vegetarian items that can be found right under your nose. If you don't see anything on the menu, ask your server what they have to offer for vegetarians.

You know I am not a vegetarian, but I have cooked for many clients who had special dietary needs and preferences. I am so happy to share some of the recipes that I have used. You'll find that these dishes are quite tasty!

Chapter 13

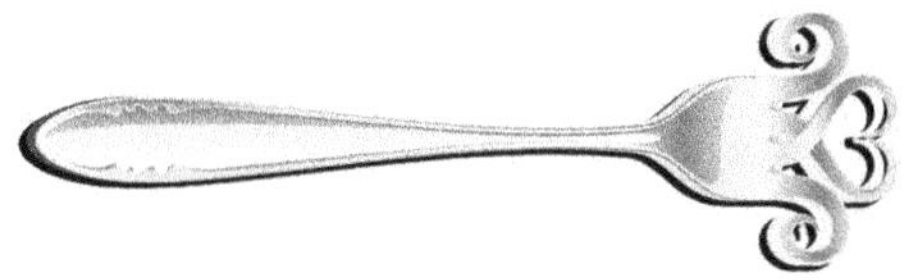

~VEGETARIAN BREAKFAST~

BERRY BAGELS

Jam:
3 cups ripe raspberries
1 cup ripe strawberries, stemmed
1/2 cup maple syrup
1/4 cup lemon juice
2 tsp. corn starch

Boil over low heat for at least 45 minutes. Cool and chill in refrigerator until ready to use.

To make spread:
3 Tbsp. tofu cream cheese
2 Tbsp. Jam mixture, chilled
2 multi-grain bagels, toasted

Make jam the night before. In the morning, whip together the tofu cream cheese and jam. Toast the bagels an spread the mixture on the hot bagels! Serves 2.

Sharon Fox

ORANGE JUICE FROSTY

4 Valencia oranges, squeezed
1 ripe banana
1/3 cup frozen peaches
1/2 cup frozen pineapple
1/3 cup ice

Put all ingredients in a blender. Blend until smooth, pour into 2 glasses and serve. Garnish with orange slices. Makes 2 servings.

FEEL LIKE ROYALTY SMOOTHIES

1 1/2 cups pink grapefruit juice, freshly squeezed if possible
3/4 cup wild blueberries
1/2 cup strawberries
1/2 cup ice
1 ripe banana (fresh or frozen)
1 kiwi, peeled
1/2 tsp. Spirulina powder (found in health food stores)

Blend all ingredients in a blender. Pour into 2 glasses and be energized for the day! Makes 2 servings.

If you prefer a thicker smoothie, peel banana, slice and freeze.

Sharon Fox

VEGETARIAN BREAKFAST BURRITOS

3-4 flour tortillas
3 Tbsp. vegetable oil
1 clove garlic, minced
1/2 onion, diced
1 lb. firm tofu, chopped in 1-inch pieces
1/2 cup sliced mushrooms
1 tomato, diced
1/8 tsp. turmeric
dash of Tabasco sauce, optional
salt and pepper to taste
non-dairy Vegan sour cream, optional
grated Vegan cheese, optional

Warm the tortillas in oven or skillet until soft. In a large skillet, heat the oil and cook the onion and garlic for a couple of minutes. add the tofu, mushrooms, and tomato and cook 4-5 minutes, stirring frequently, until mushrooms are soft. Remove from heat and add turmeric and a little Tabasco, if you are using it. Season with salt and pepper to taste. Divide mixture between 3-4 tortillas and top with Vegan sour cream and cheese. Wrap and serve hot.

NOTES

NOTES

Chapter 14

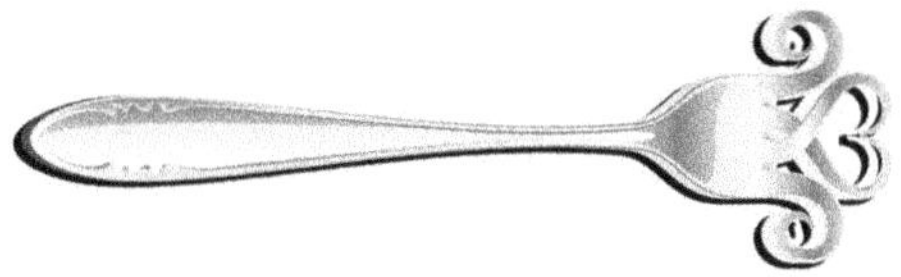

~VEGETARIAN APPETIZERS AND SNACKS~

ZESTY ONION-TOMATO DIP

8 oz. cream cheese, softened
1/2 of a large tomato, diced
1 clove garlic, minced
1/3 of an onion, diced
1 Tbsp. hot sauce
1 Tbsp. sweet paprika

chips for dipping

Combine all dip ingredients together in a bowl. Stir to combine well and serve or chill until ready to serve. Makes 1 1/2 cups.

COLORFUL POMEGRANATE AND PERSIMMON SALAD

8 cups baby spinach leaves
3 persimmons, cut into thin slices
1 red onion, thinly sliced
3 Tbsp. sherry vinegar
7 Tbsp. olive oil
salt and pepper
seeds from 1 large pomegranate

In a large bowl, combine the spinach, persimmons, and onion slices. In a small bowl, whisk together the vinegar and oil. Toss with the salad. Add salt and pepper to taste. Sprinkle the pomegranate seeds and serve. Makes 8 servings.

ELEGANT CARROT-THYME SOUP

2 Tbsp. extra-virgin olive oil
1 bag of carrots, peeled and chopped
1 cup chopped yellow onion
1 1/2 Tbsp. chopped fresh thyme, some for garnish
3 cups vegetable broth
1 cup water
1 Tbsp. brown sugar
1 tsp. black pepper
1 tsp. salt
1 cup sour cream, for garnish

Heat oil in a skillet over medium heat. Cook the carrots and onions for 15-20 minutes, stirring frequently, until carrots are soft. Add 1 Tbsp. thyme, salt, and pepper. Remove from heat and allow to cool for about 5 minutes. Add the mixture to a blender with brown sugar and one cup of the vegetable broth. Blend until smooth. Add remaining broth one cup at a time until you reach the desired consistency. Blend until it reaches a butternut squash color. Pour into a 10 quart pot and heat. Add salt and pepper to taste. If it's too thick, add a little water. Ladle hot soup into bowls and spoon a dollop of sour cream into the center. Sprinkle with a little of the remaining thyme for garnish. Makes 6-8 servings.

FRUIT SALSA AND CINNAMON CHIPS

2 kiwis, peeled and diced
2 apples, diced
8 oz. fresh raspberries
1 lb. strawberries
2 Tbsp. sugar
1 Tbsp. brown sugar
3 Tbsp. your favorite preserves
10 10-inch flour tortillas
butter flavor cooking spray
2 Tbsp. sugar-cinnamon

Mix the kiwis, apples, raspberries, strawberries, sugar, brown sugar, and preserves in a large mixing bowl. Cover and chill 20 minutes.

Preheat your oven to 350 degrees. Coat one side of each tortilla with cooking spray. Cut into wedges and place on a cookie sheet. Sprinkle with cinnamon-sugar. Spray again with cooking spray and bake 8-10 minutes, until they begin to brown. Allow them to cool for about 15 minutes before serving. Serve with chilled fruit salsa. Makes 10 servings.

NOTES

NOTES

Chapter 15

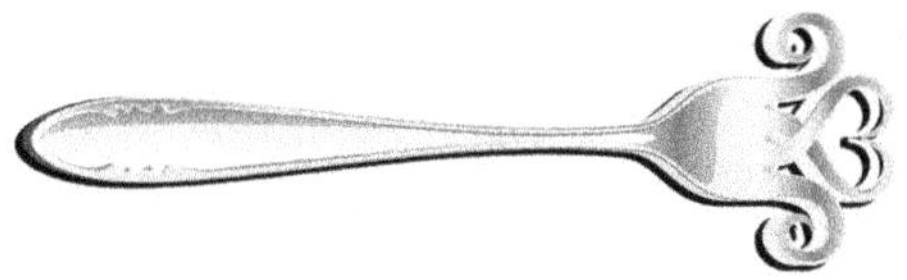

~VEGETARIAN MEALS~

SAUTEED RED CABBAGE

1/2 of a red cabbage, shredded
1 chopped apple
1 small onion, chopped
1/2 cup water
1/2 cup raisins
1/2 tsp. cinnamon

Heat a non-stick pan over medium heat. Add all ingredients, stirring occasionally. Cook for about 10-12 minutes. Makes 4 servings.

Sharon Fox

POTATOES, CABBAGE, AND PEAS WITH RICE

2 cups rice
4 cups water
5 medium size potatoes, peeled and thinly sliced
2 cups water
1/2 of a green cabbage
10 oz. fresh or frozen peas
2 tsp. curry powder
1 tsp. turmeric
1/2 tsp. ginger
1/2 tsp. garlic powder
1/8 tsp. cayenne pepper
salt to taste (optional)

Cook the rice in 4 cups of water in a covered pot over medium-high heat until tender. In a separate pan, add the sliced potatoes to 2 cups of water and heat over medium-high heat. Shred the cabbage and add to the potatoes. Add peas and spices. Cover and continue cooking, stirring occasionally until potatoes are done. Serve over the rice. Makes 6 servings.

VEGETABLE TAGINE WITH HARISSA YOGURT SAUCE

Yogurt Sauce:
8 oz. Greek yogurt
1 Tbsp. extra-virgin olive oil
1 tsp. Harissa sauce (hot chili sauce)
1 clove garlic, minced
coarse Kosher sauce, to taste

Vegetable Tagine:
Kosher salt
1 lb. carrots, peeled and cut into 1/2 inch pieces
1 3/4 lb. turnip, peeled and cut into 1/2 inch pieces
3 Tbsp. butter
1 3/4 cups green onions, chopped
2 Tbsp. Italian parsley, chopped
2 Tbsp. fresh mint, chopped
2 cloves garlic, minced
1 tsp. paprika
1 tsp. cumin
1/2 tsp. ground coriander
1/2 cup dry white wine
2 tsp. all purpose flour
1 can (15 oz.) chick peas, drained and rinsed
5 oz. bag baby spinach
1-3 Tbsp. fresh lemon juice

Make the sauce by mixing all the ingredients. Cover and chill. Bring 8 cups water to boil in a heavy saucepan. Sprinkle in some salt and add the carrots. Cook until tender., about 4 minutes. Use a slotted spoon to transfer the carrots to a large bowl of ice water to stop the cooking process. Return the water to boil. Add the turnip and cook until tender. Remove the cooked turnips and put them in the bowl with the carrots. Reserve the cooking liquid. Melt butter in a large heavy pot over medium heat. Add next seven ingredients. Sprinkle with salt and pepper. Cook about 8 minutes until onions are soft. Add wine and simmer until reduced by half, about 5 minutes. Stir in flour. add the carrots, turnips, beans, spinach, and 2 cups of the reserved cooking liquid. Bring to a simmer and cook until hot. Add more liquid if needed. Season to taste with salt, pepper, and lemon juice. Serve with a dollop of the yogurt sauce on top. Makes 6 servings.

OPEN FACED RATAOUILLE SANDWICH

1 small eggplant, sliced into 1-inch slices
1 small zucchini or yellow summer squash, sliced into 3/4-inch slices
1 red bell pepper, cut into strips
1/2 of a small red onion, cut into 1/2-inch wedges
1 Tbsp. olive oil
1/2 tsp. herbs de Provence (found in spice section of grocery store)
6 cherry tomatoes, cut in half
4 slices (1/2-inch thick) bakery fresh artisan bread
1 clove roasted garlic, cut in half
2 Tbsp. balsamic vinegar
4 slices provolone cheese
fresh thyme sprigs, for garnish (optional)

Preheat your oven to 400 degrees. Coat a large shallow roasting pan with cooking spray. Add eggplant, zucchini, red pepper, and onion to the pan. Drizzle with olive oil and sprinkle with herbs of Provence, 1/8 tsp. salt, and 1/8 tsp. black pepper. Toss to coat veggies. Roast in oven for about 30 minutes, tossing once after first 15 minutes. Add the tomatoes and roast 15-20 minutes longer, until veggies are tender and some are lightly browned.
In the meantime, rub the bread slices with the cut side of the garlic clove. Place one slice of bread on each of four serving plates. Sprinkle balsamic vinegar over the veggies and toss gently to coat. Spoon the warm veggies on bread. (Garnish with fresh thyme sprigs.) Cover each one with a slice of cheese and return to oven until bread is toasted and the cheese is melted, about 5 minutes. Makes 4 open faced sandwiches.

STUFFED ACORN SQUASH

1 baked acorn squash (to bake, cut in half, scoop out the seeds, place face down in a glass casserole dish. Add enough water to just cover the bottom of pan and bake at 350 degrees for 35 minutes)

1 cup broccoli florets, chopped
1/2 of a red bell pepper, chopped
4 sliced mushrooms
1/4 cup water
1 cup cooked chickpeas
2 Tbsp. balsamic vinaigrette
crumbled feta cheese
salt and pepper

In a medium non-stick pan, cook and stir all of the veggies in 1/4 cup of water for about 4-5 minutes, until tender. Add the chickpeas and simmer on low heat until the chickpeas are heated through. Pour 2 Tbsp. of the vinaigrette in with the veggies and toss gently. Divide the vegetable mixture in half and stuff each half of the baked acorn squash. Crumble the desired amount of feta cheese on top and season with salt and pepper to taste.

POTATO CURRY WITH SWISS CHARD

1 lb. Swiss chard, chop leaves into 2-inch pieces, cut stalks into 1-inch pieces
2 Tbsp. sunflower oil
1 onion, thinly sliced
3 cloves garlic, peeled
1 jalapeno, seeded and chopped finely
1 small piece ginger (1 inch), peeled and chopped
1 tsp, Garam Masala (Indian spice found in spice section of grocery
1/2 tsp. mustard seeds
1/2 tsp. cumin
1/4 tsp. turmeric
3 cardamom pods, crushed
3/4 lb. new potatoes, quartered
1 cup plain yogurt
1 1/2 Tbsp. tomato puree
1 small bunch of coriander, chopped
1 small handful toasted almonds, chopped
sea salt and black pepper

Heat oil in a large saucepan over medium heat and cook onion until barely golden. Meanwhile pound the jalapeno, garlic, and ginger together with a pinch of salt to make a paste. Add this to the onion and cook for 2 minutes. Add remaining spices and cook for 1-2 minutes. Add the potatoes and Swiss chard stalks and cook for 4-5 minutes, stirring frequently to coat evenly with spices. Stir in enough water to just cover the veggies. Bring to a simmer, cover and cook for about 12 minutes, until potatoes are just tender. Add the chard leaves, stir and cook until wilted.

In a bowl, whisk together the yogurt, tomato puree, and some of the hot liquid from the pot. Remove curry from heat and add the yogurt mixture. Stir to combine and return to heat to warm through very gently. Do not allow to boil or the yogurt will curdle. Stir in most of the coriander. Taste and season with salt and pepper if needed. Top with remaining coriander and toasted nuts. Serve with brown rice and your choice of bread.

NOTES

Chapter 16

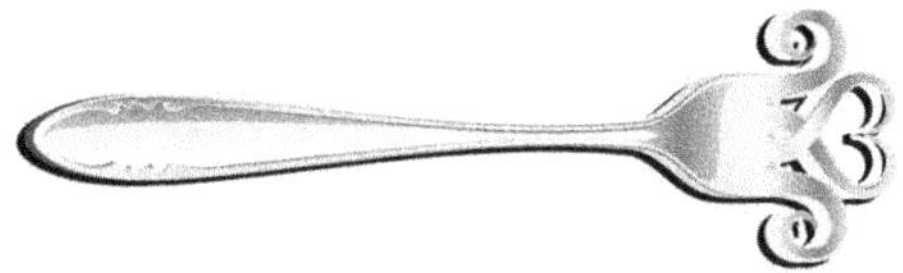

~VEGETARIAN DESSERTS~

VEGAN RAW FRUIT COBBLER

Crumb topping:
1 1/2 cups shredded coconut
1 1/2 cups toasted walnuts or dehydrated to make them dry and crispy
1/2 tsp. salt
1/3 cup pitted dates

Filling:
3 cups frozen cherries, thawed and drained
1/2 cup pitted dates
2 tsp. lemon juice
1/8 tsp. cinnamon

To make topping, put all ingredients in food processor except the dates. Process to make coarse crumbs, add dates one at a time.
To make the filling, in a blender combine 1 cup cherries with dates, lemon juice, and cinnamon. Toss in a bowl with remaining 2 cups cherries. Put cherry mixture into 3 serving dishes and top with the crumb topping.

You may also use frozen blueberries or strawberries.

Sharon Fox

VEGAN CHOCOLATE CREAM PIE

Crust:
5 oz. all-natural chocolate snap cookies, broken into pieces
2 Tbsp. cocoa powder
2 Tbsp. canola oil

Filling:
1 can coconut milk
1/4 cup cornstarch
1/3 cup plus 1 Tbsp. vegan chocolate chips
1 tsp. vanilla extract
1/3 cup sugar
pinch of salt
8 oz. tofu (non-dairy) cream cheese

Make Crust:
Preheat oven to 350 degrees. In a food processor, pulse the cookie pieces and cocoa powder until fine crumbs are formed. Transfer to a bowl and add oil. Stir to combine and then press into a 9-inch pie pan using a glass to get the crust even and up the sides. Chill for 20 minutes and then bake for 10 minutes, until set. Cool on a wire rack.

Make Filling:
Shake the can of coconut milk before opening. Add the cornstarch to about 1/4 cup of the coconut milk and whisk until smooth. In a medium size saucepan, combine the cornstarch mixture, remaining coconut milk, vanilla, and sugar over medium heat. as it begins to heat, add the chocolate chips and bring to a simmer, stirring frequently and don't allow to boil. Cook gently until it thickens and has a pudding consistency. Pour into a large bowl and add the tofu cream cheese. Stir well until completely incorporated. Pour into cooled crust and refrigerate overnight or at least 5 hours. Serve as is or with a non-dairy whipped topping.

COCONUT PUDDING

1 1/2 cup coconut milk
2/3 cup powdered sugar
1/3 cup cornstarch
1 tsp. vanilla
cinnamon and fruit for garnish, optional

In a small saucepan, over medium-low heat, combine all ingredients. Stir constantly and cook for about 6-8 minutes until creamy, smooth and slightly thickened. Pour into serving dishes and chill in refrigerator to set. You may want to cover with plastic wrap on the surface to prevent skin from forming. Garnish with cinnamon and fresh fruit before serving.

Sharon Fox

VEGAN OATMEAL-CRANBERRY COOKIES

3/4 cup margarine
1/3 cup sugar
3/4 cup brown sugar
1 tsp. vanilla
1/2 cup soy milk
1 cup flour
1/2 tsp. baking soda
1/4 tsp. ground ginger
1/4 tsp. ground cloves
1/2 tsp. cinnamon
1/4 tsp. nutmeg
3 cups rolled oats
1 cup dried cranberries (Craisins)

Cream together the margarine and sugars until smooth. Add vanilla and soy milk and combine well. Sift together dry ingredients and add to batter slowly. Mix well and then stir in the cranberries. Chill for at least 30 minutes. Preheat oven to 350 degrees. Spoon 1 1/2-inch balls onto ungreased cookie sheet and bake 10-15 minutes. Enjoy!

NOTES

NOTES

Chapter 17

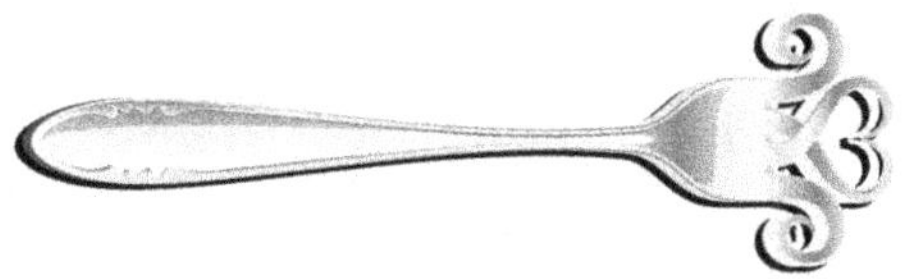

~ABOUT GOING GLUTEN-FREE~

If you are familiar with the gluten-free diet, you know that regular breads, bagels, muffins, and many other store-bought baked goods are off limits. There are a few things you need to know before you purchase gluten-free grain products or make them at home.

What is Gluten?

Gluten is actually a protein present in wheat flour, which is also widely used in commercial and homemade baked goods. It's also found in flour made from barley, rye, spelt, and triticale, a cross between wheat and rye. Other products include: white flour, graham flour, semolina, wheat germ, and wheat bran. Gluten helps dough to rise and lends shape and a chewy texture to baked goods. Baked goods are not the only foods that may contain gluten.

Foods that contain gluten.

Many convenience foods that you pick up everyday contain gluten. You may be surprised to know that some of these items have gluten: pasta, couscous, flour tortillas, pastries, cereals, crackers, beer, gravy, dressings, sauces. Others that may be more surprising include: broth in soups and bouillon cubes, imitation fish, lunch meat and hot dogs, most chips and candy, self-basting turkey, soy sauce, and frozen fried foods.

There are over 3 million Americans who are sensitive to gluten (gluten intolerant) or have Celiac Disease. Many people now are slowly reducing gluten from their diets. Finding gluten-free products is much easier now than over ten years ago. These products may also taste better today than they did in the past, but they aren't necessarily more nutritious. It is very important to read the labels on all products before purchasing, especially if you are on a special diet. You don't want to sacrifice vitamins and minerals.

Purchase gluten-free products with added vitamins and minerals, and always look for items made with whole grain flour or bean flour to help you get the nutrients you need. Although there is no shortage of carbohydrates in most gluten-free baked goods, most are lower in fiber. When there is no gluten in a recipe, it takes far more gluten-free ingredients to produce a tasty product.

The refined carbohydrates typically used in gluten-free products and mixes, including white rice flour and tapioca, produce baked goods that are much higher in calories and total carbohydrates than regular versions. Simply swapping regular bread and other baked goods with gluten-free products without any regard for calories can easily lead to weight gain! Gluten-free products won't necessarily help you with weight control, and they may actually hinder your efforts to lose weight if you're not very careful. For this reason, you should always check the labels for calorie counts per serving and stick to serving size portions.

Gluten-Free Home Baking

When you're baking at home, it is impossible to simply substitute gluten-free flours for those with gluten and get the same results. Baking is a science and you really need to use gluten-free recipes for perfect results. There is a large variety of gluten-free flours on the market. They are made from brown rice, white beans, potato, and oats.

If you aren't experienced with mixing flours to create a blend that you can use all the time, it's best to purchase a pre-mixed gluten-free blend. Having a good flour blend on hand at all times will make your baking experience so much easier. Here is a great homemade blend that you may want to keep on hand:

1 1/2 cups sorghum or brown rice flour
1 1/2 cups potato starch or cornstarch
1 cup tapioca flour

Whisk together and store in a cool, dry place. When substituting this blend for wheat flour in recipes, measure it as though it were wheat flour.

Celiac Disease, Gluten Sensitivity, Gluten-Free Dieting

In 2008, Oprah Winfrey temporarily gave up gluten as part of a 21-day cleanse diet. Over the past 15 years or so, going gluten-free has become a way of boosting health and energy, coping with ADHD, autism, headaches, and other conditions. But there are certain people who actually need this gluten-free diet. Long before the gluten-free diet was a popular fad diet, it was tested to be a proven treatment for Celiac Disease or Gluten Sensitivity.

Celiac Disease is an autoimmune disease in which a person cannot tolerate gluten. If a person with this disease eats gluten, the lining of their small intestine becomes inflamed and damaged. That hampers the absorption of nutrients and can lead to malnutrition and weight loss. Celiac patients also struggle with distressing symptoms, such as diarrhea, stomach upset, abdominal pain, and bloating. In some cases, Celiac Disease may take several years to diagnose because doctors mistake it for irritable bowel syndrome or other diseases.

Some people may test negative for Celiac Disease and may have a condition called "gluten-sensitivity". In this case, the intestine isn't damaged but all other symptoms may be present in addition to fatigue and headaches. About 1-2% of the American population are sensitive to gluten. The rate of this disease is rising, doubling every 20 years.

Testing

Celiac Disease can be diagnosed through a blood test and an intestinal biopsy that shows the damage to the intestine, but there is no reliable test for gluten sensitivity as of yet. To diagnose gluten sensitivity, the doctor will have to go by the symptoms the patient tell him about when eating certain foods that contain gluten. If you think you may be sensitive to gluten, see your doctor for testing and keep track of all your symptoms. Share all this information a your doctor visit. Remember, for the blood test to be accurate for Celiac Disease, you must actually have gluten in your system.

Gluten-Free Lifestyle

Having Celiac Disease means that you will need to follow a gluten-free diet for the rest of your life. Permanently following a strict diet can be difficult, especially if you don't have any symptoms. But the intestinal damage will still occur when you eat foods with gluten, regardless of whether you notice any symptoms. The following strategies will help you stick to your gluten-free diet:

- ❖ Seek guidance from a registered dietitian or other health professionals for ways to find and cook gluten-free meals. Keep a food diary until you are familiar with a healthy menu and variety that works for you.

- Be aware of foods that may contain hidden gluten. Always read the labels of processed foods carefully. "Hydrolyzed vegetable protein" may come from wheat and contain gluten.
- Keep your gluten-free flour, counter tops, utensils, and appliances clean before using. Use a separate toaster for regular breads and gluten-free breads.
- When eating out, let the server know about your special diet to avoid gluten products on your plate.
- Eat plenty of fresh fruits and vegetables to avoid constipation

Children and teens may have other issues dealing with Celiac Disease. They don't want to feel different from their friends. Help them to realize that their intestines will be damaged if they continue to eat gluten products. There are several strategies to help your child stick to their special diet:

- Contact your local hospital or doctor for support groups in your area. They will offer great ideas and answer many of your concerns.
- Talk to your child's teachers or school nurse about healthy diet at school.
- Allow your child to pick out some of their favorite meal items and have them readily available.
- Teach your child to prepare some fun snacks or dishes and serve them when their friends are there. When their friends enjoy these treats, they will feel more comfortable eating them as well.

Family counseling will be very helpful for managing the emotional challenges that may come with a new lifestyle.

Remember to explore new recipes, try new foods, and work together as a family to encourage healthier eating.

One very important tip to always remember if you are cooking for a gluten-intolerant or Celiac Disease patient:

ALWAYS be sure that all utensils, supplies, and counter tops are clean. Any flour or gluten residue from other foods can easily be picked up into your food.

Chapter 18

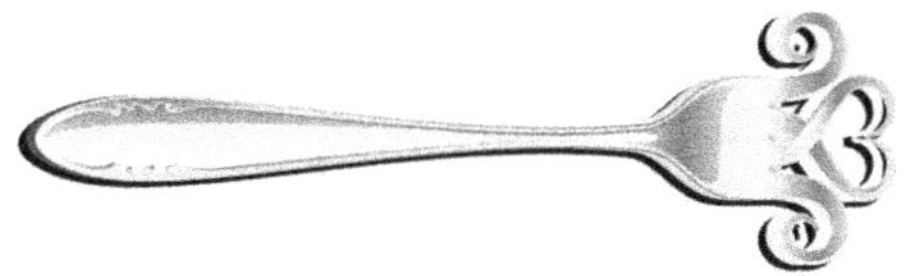

~GLUTEN-FREE BREAKFAST~

GLUTEN-FREE BUTTERMILK PANCAKES

1 1/4 cup gluten-free flour blend (with added xanathan gum)
2 Tbsp. cane sugar
1 tsp. gluten-free baking powder
1 tsp. baking soda
1/4 tsp. salt
1 1/4 cup buttermilk
2 Tbsp. vegetable oil
1 egg
1/2 tsp. gluten-free-vanilla extract

Combine all dry ingredients in a mixing bowl and mix well. In a separate bowl, combine the buttermilk, oil, egg, and vanilla. Mix well and stir into the dry mixture. If the batter seem too thick, add a little buttermilk one teaspoon at a time.
Heat your griddle or skillet over medium heat. Lightly brush the surface with oil. Pour 1/4 cup for each pancake and cook until golden brown on both sides. Makes about 6 pancakes.

Note: If your gluten-free flour doesn't contain added xanathan gum, add 1 tsp. to the recipe)

GLUTEN-FREE OVERNIGHT WAFFLES

2 1/4 cups milk or your favorite milk substitute
1 pkg. dry yeast
1 tsp. sugar
1 tsp. salt
1 stick butter
2 cups gluten-free all purpose flour mix
2 eggs, beaten well
1/4 tsp. baking soda
2 tsp. vanilla extract

Warm the milk and butter in saucepan just until butter melts. When it cools to lukewarm (105 degrees), add the yeast and sugar and let sit until the yeast is bubbly. This should take about 5 minutes. Pour the liquid into a container with a tight fitting lid (a pitcher works out wonderfully!).
Add salt and flour mix and whisk until smooth. Cover tightly and keep at room temperature overnight. Don't refrigerate. When you are ready to cook the waffles, stir in the beaten eggs, baking soda, and vanilla. Pour about 1/2 cup for each waffle into the waffle iron. Cook until golden brown. Store unused batter in refrigerator up to 3 days in refrigerator. Makes 6-8 waffles.

GLUTEN-FREE FRENCH TOAST

8 slices of your favorite gluten-free bread
4 beaten eggs
1/2 to 3/4 cup milk (or canned organic coconut milk)
1 tsp. sugar or honey
pinch of salt
1 tsp. vanilla extract
canola oil for frying
1 Tbsp. gluten-free powdered sugar

Combine eggs, milk, sugar, salt, and vanilla in a shallow bowl and mix well. Dip bread slices in mixture on both sides, allowing it to soak up the egg mixture. Brush surface of griddle or skillet with oil and heat over medium-high heat. Lay soaked bread slices on hot griddle and cook until golden on both sides. Serve with butter and a dusting of powdered sugar (gluten-free). Makes 8 slices, 4 servings.

GLUTEN-FREE OVERNIGHT OATMEAL

1 cup gluten-free rolled oats
1 cup warm water
2 Tbsp. lemon juice
1/2 tsp. salt

When you are ready to cook the oatmeal, you'll need:
1 cup water
1/2 cup raisins
1/4 tsp. cinnamon

Complete Directions:

Pour 1 cup warm water mixed with 2 Tbsp. lemon juice in a wide-mouth jar. Add oats and stir and put the lid on the jar. Allow to sit in a warm place overnight. In the morning place the soaked oats, 1 cup water, salt, and raisins in a medium saucepan. Cook over low heat about 3 minutes. Remove heat and stir in cinnamon and allow to stand about 5 minutes. Serve with honey, maple syrup, or your favorite sweetener. Makes 4 servings.

GLUTEN-FREE EGSS BENEDICT

4 gluten-free English muffins, sliced in half

Sauce:
4 Tbsp. butter or light olive oil
4 Tbsp. rice flour
1 cup milk or canned organic coconut milk
2 large egg yolks
2 Tbsp. melted butter
3 Tbsp. fresh squeezed lemon juice
salt and pepper
dash of Tabasco sauce
8 poached eggs
8 slices gluten-free deli ham

Place 4 Tbsp. butter or light olive oil in heavy saucepan and melt over low heat. Whisk in the rice flour until smooth. Season to taste with salt and pepper. Remove from heat and whisk in milk and then return to heat. Continue to whisk until it comes to a boil. Remove from heat and whisk in yolks one at a time, very quickly to prevent scrambling. Return to low heat. Whisk in melted butter, lemon juice, and Tabasco sauce. Remove from heat. You don't want the sauce to be too thick. If you need to thin it out a bit, just add a few drops of hot water.
To serve, toast eh split English muffins in toaster. While they are toasting, heat ham slices in small skillet to heat through. Butter the English muffins and fold 2 slices of ham on each piece of bread. Top each with a poached egg and spoon about 3-4 Tbsp. of the Hollandaise sauce over the top.

To poach eggs:

Fresh eggs
1-2 tsp. vinegar

Bring a saucepan half filled with water almost to a boil. Don't let it come to a full boil. Add vinegar. Crack eggs one at a time into a bowl and gently slide them into water. Only cook 1-2 at a time. Nudge the whites closer to the yolk until they begin to firm up. Turn off heat and cover for 4 minutes. Remove with a slotted spoon. You can use the ring of a mason jar to mold the eggs if you prefer. Just lay the ring into the pan. Slide the raw egg into the ring!

GLUTEN-FREE BANANA-VANILLA SMOOTHIE

2 cups rice or almond milk or canned organic coconut milk, cold
1 peeled, sliced banana (frozen after you slice it)
1 tsp. vanilla extract
dash of nutmeg, optional

Pour milk into blender. Add banana slices and vanilla. Blend until smooth. Pour into 2 glasses and garnish with nutmeg. Serve. Makes 2 servings.

HIGH PROTEIN STRAWBERRY FLAX SMOOTHIE

1/2 cup good fat-free Greek yogurt
1/2 cup frozen strawberries
1 Tbsp. freshly ground golden flax seeds
1 tsp. vanilla extract
1/8 to 1/4 tsp. Stevia or sugar
1/2 cup cold spring water

Put all ingredients in blender and pulse until smooth. Pour into 12oz. glass and enjoy! Makes one good serving.

GLUTEN-FREE APPLE OAT MUFFINS

2 cups freshly ground gluten free rolled oats
2 tsp. gluten-free baking powder
1/4 tsp. baking soda
1 1/2 tsp. cinnamon
1/4 cup dark brown sugar
1/4 cup gluten free plain yogurt
1/2 cup 100% apple juice
2 eggs and 1 egg white, slightly beaten
4 Tbsp. canola oil
1/2 tsp. vanilla
1 cup shredded fresh apple (do not peel the apple)
1/2 cup chopped walnuts

Topping:
1 Tbsp. sugar mixed with 1/2 tsp. cinnamon

Preheat your oven to 350 degrees. Pulse the oats in a clean grinder or food processor until a soft oat flour is created. Place the oat flour, baking powder, baking soda, brown sugar, and cinnamon in a mixing bowl and stir to combine. Lightly beat the eggs in a small bowl. Add the yogurt, apple juice, oil, and vanilla. Whisk to blend well and pour into the dry ingredients. Stir to mix well. Fold in the shredded apples and walnuts. Line muffin pan with cupcake liners and fill each cup 3/4 full. Bake for about 16-18 minutes, until toothpick inserted in center comes out clean. Sprinkle the hot muffins with sugar/cinnamon mixture. Cool for 15 minutes before serving.

GLUTEN-FREE TROPICAL MORNING MUFFINS

1 1/4 cups sugar
2 1/4 cups gluten-free all purpose flour (with xanathan gum added)
1 Tbsp. cinnamon
2 tsp. baking soda
1 tsp. baking powder
1/2 tsp. salt
2 cups grated carrots
1 large, peeled shredded apple
8 oz. crushed pineapple, drained
3/4 cup raisins
1/2 cup shredded, sweetened coconut
1/2 cup chopped walnuts or pecans
3 large eggs
1 cup canola oil
1 1/2 tsp. vanilla

NOTE: If your gluten-free flour doesn't contain gum, add 1 tsp. xanathan gum with the flour.

Preheat your oven to 350 degrees. Line a muffin pan with cupcake liners. In a large mixing bowl, combine sugar, gluten-free flour blend, cinnamon, baking soda, baking powder, and salt. Whisk together to mix well. In a separate bowl, combine shredded carrots, apples, pineapple, raisins, coconut, and nuts. Stir to mix well. Add the fruit mixture to dry mixture. Add eggs, oil, and vanilla. Beat well to combine all ingredients. Fill the muffin cups about 3/4 full. Bake 25-30 minutes until done. Makes about 24 muffins.

NOTES

NOTES

Chapter 19

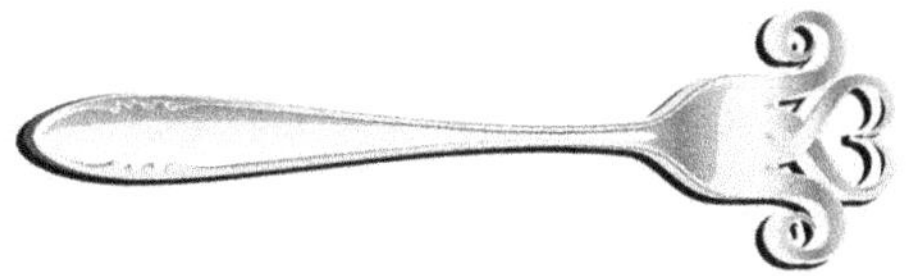

~APPETIZERS, SNACKS, AND SALADS~

LOBSTER FRITTERS

vegetable oil, for frying
1 cup gluten-free pancake mix
1/2 cup finely chopped onions
1/2 cup finely chopped celery
1/2 cup unsweetened shredded coconut
1/2 cup crushed gluten free crackers
1 lobster tail, cleaned and chopped
1 Tbsp. Old Bay seasoning
1 1/4 tsp. baking powder
1 tsp. salt
1 tsp. black pepper
2 eggs
1/2 cup evaporated milk
1 Tbsp. garlic butter, melted

Heat oil in iron skillet or deep fryer to 365 degrees. Combine the gluten free pancake mix, onions, celery, coconut, crushed crackers, lobster, Old Bay, baking powder, salt, and pepper in a bowl. In a separate bowl, combine eggs, milk, and garlic butter. Stir egg mixture into dry mixture to make a batter. Drop by rounded Tablespoons into hot oil and fry until golden brown, about 3 minutes. Remove and drain on paper towels. Serve with your favorite dipping sauce. Makes 6 servings.

Sharon Fox

ROMAN STUFFED DATE APPETIZERS

12 pitted dates
1/4 cup toasted pine nuts, chopped
3 Tbsp. red wine
fresh cracked black pepper
1/4 cup honey or real maple syrup

Stuff the dates with chopped nuts. Insert in the space left by the pit. Place in a non-stick saucepan. Sprinkle with pepper. Add wine then drizzle with honey or maple syrup. Cook over medium-low heat, until the skins begin to peel off naturally. Transfer to a serving plate and serve warm. Great for parties! Makes 4 servings.

If you have problems with these sticking, you can place them in a baking pan lined with parchment paper, sprayed with cooking spray to prevent sticking. Bake at 375 until skins begin to peel off fruit.

GLUTEN FREE MACHO-NACHOS

12 oz. gluten free corn tortilla chips
1 lb. lean ground beef
2 Tbsp. gluten free taco seasoning, homemade recipe follows
6 cups shredded cheddar, Monterey jack blend cheeses
1/2 cup chopped yellow onion
1/2 cup red or orange bell pepper, chopped
1/2 cup pickled jalapenos, sliced and pat dry
1/2 cup sliced black olives
1/2 cup sliced green onions
1/2 cup Roma tomatoes, seeded and chopped
1/4 cup chopped parsley or cilantro

Brown beef in heavy pan and drain off fat. Add the taco seasoning and set aside. heat your oven to 400 degrees. In a 9x13-inch pan, spread 1/3 of the chips. Top with 1/3 of the meat then 1/3 of each: onion, bell pepper, jalapenos, black olives, green onions, and tomatoes. Top with 1/3 of the cheese. Repeat two more times until finished. Bake for 20 minutes until cheese melts. Sprinkle the parsley or cilantro over the top before serving. Makes 8 appetizer servings.

BONUS RECIPE:

Gluten-free taco seasoning:

2 Tbsp. gluten free onion powder
2 tsp. gluten free garlic powder
1 Tbsp. salt
1 Tbsp. chili powder
1 1/2 tsp. crushed red pepper
1 1/2 tsp. gluten free ground cumin
1 tsp. dried oregano
1 1/2 tsp. cornstarch

Put all ingredients in a clean dry 8 oz. jar with tight fitting lid. Shake to combine.

Sharon Fox

GLUTEN-FREE TURKEY SALAD

1 5 oz. pkg. ready-to-eat leafy greens
8 oz. julienne sliced deli turkey (cut in strips)
1 bottle gluten-free poppy seed salad dressing (or your favorite)
1 cup gluten-free croutons
1/4 cup Parmesan cheese, optional

Divide greens among 4 plates. Top with 2 oz. turkey, croutons, cheese, and dressing. Serves 4.

SPINACH SALAD WITH HOMEMADE FRENCH DRESSING

1 lb. fresh spinach leaved, washed and dried
4 slices cooked gluten-free bacon, crumbled
3 hard boiled eggs, chopped
1 cup red onions, thinly sliced
1 cup mushrooms, thinly sliced
1/4 tsp. smoked paprika
gluten free French Dressing

Tear spinach leaves into bite-size pieces. Toss with bacon, sliced mushrooms, and onion slices. Top with chopped boiled eggs and sprinkle with paprika. Makes 4-6 servings.

Gluten-Free French Dressing:

1 cup extra virgin olive oil
1/2 to 3/4 cup sugar (according to desired sweetness)
1/3 cup gluten-free ketchup
1/4 cup apple cider vinegar
1 tsp. Worcestershire sauce

Whisk all ingredients together until sugar dissolves and dressing is glossy. Pour into a jar with tight fitting lid. Store in refrigerator. Makes 1 pint.

GLUTEN-FREE POTATO SALAD

6 medium Russet potatoes, cubed in 1 1/2 inch cubes
1 tsp. salt, for cooking potatoes
1 cup chopped celery
1/2 cup chopped yellow onions
3 green onions, sliced
1/2 cup chopped parsley
3 hard boiled eggs, chopped
1 cup mayonnaise
2 Tbsp. apple cider vinegar
1 Tbsp. prepared mustard
2 tsp. sugar
2 tsp. celery seed
1 1/2 tsp. salt
1/2 tsp. white pepper
1/2 tsp. paprika, for garnish

Peel potatoes and cube. Cook in boiling salted water for 30-35 minutes, until tender. Drain and cool. In a large mixing bowl, whisk together the mayonnaise, vinegar, mustard, sugar, salt, celery seed, and white pepper. Fold the celery, onions, and eggs into the potatoes. Pour the dressing over the potato mixture and gently stir to combine. Chill in refrigerator until ready to serve. Sprinkle a little paprika over the top before serving. Makes 8 servings.

COLORFUL COLESLAW W/ SESAME DRESSING

8 cups red cabbage, thinly sliced
8 medium carrots, shredded
6 green onions, thinly sliced
1/4 cup red bell pepper, diced
1/4 cup green bell peppers, diced
1/2 cup sliced green olives with pimentos
2 tsp. celery seed
1 tsp. salt
black pepper to taste

Gluten-Free Vinaigrette:
3/4 cup light olive oil
2 tsp. toasted sesame oil
1 Tbsp. cane sugar
1/4 cup rice wine vinegar
salt and pepper to taste

Wash and prepare all slaw veggies and put them in a large bowl. Toss to combine. Add salt and pepper and celery seed. Mix well. Makes 8 servings.

For the dressing: Place the olive oil, sesame oil, vinegar, sugar, salt and pepper in a blender. Pulse for about 10 seconds to mix well. Pour into jar and cover with lid. Chill until ready to use.

BLACK BEAN AND CORN SALAD

2 cans black beans, drained and rinsed
2 cans black-eyed peas, drained
1 can whole corn, drained
1 large sweet onion, diced
1 bell pepper, chopped
4 garlic cloves, minced
2/3 cup apple cider vinegar
1/2 cup olive oil
1 tsp. red pepper flakes
2 tsp. sugar
1 tsp. salt
1/4 cup fresh cilantro, minced

In a medium bowl, combine black beans, peas, bell pepper, and garlic. To make the dressing, place vinegar, olive oil, red pepper flakes, sugar, and salt in a bowl and whisk to blend together. Pour dressing over veggies. Add the cilantro and stir to combine. Chill until ready to serve. Makes 8 servings.

GLUTEN-FREE POTATO CHIPS

1 large Russet potato, scrubbed clean, dried and sliced really thin
1/2 tsp. olive oil
salt, garlic salt, or barbeque seasoning

Pour oil into a plastic zip-lock bag along with the seasoning. Add the sliced potato to the bag, blow up the bag and zip to close. Shake the bag to coat potatoes well. Arrange in a single layer on a microwave-safe plate. Microwave on high for 4 minutes. Turn the chips over and arrange neatly on plate again. Cook for 2 more minutes. Watch carefully, turn and cook 2 more minutes. They will start browning. They need to brown in some places in order to crisp up nicely. Remove and place on paper towel to cool. They will crisp as they cool. Makes 1 serving for each whole potato. Enjoy!

Sharon Fox

SMOKED SALMON AND FINGERLING POTATOES

12 fingerling potatoes, cut lengthwise
1 1/2 Tbsp. extra virgin olive oil
4 oz. thinly sliced smoked salmon
1/2 cup sour cream
1 Tbsp. caviar or capers
cracked black pepper

Toss potatoes in oil to coat. Place on a rimmed baking sheet. Bake in a preheated 425 degree oven for about 20 minutes until golden brown. Let cool. Arrange pieces of smoked salmon on potatoes and top with a dollop of sour cream and a sprinkling of caviar or capers. Sprinkle with cracked black pepper. Makes 2 dozen appetizers.

KALE CHIPS

10 1/2 oz. trimmed, curly kale (about 14 cups) torn into 2-inch pieces
1 Tbsp. olive oil
salt

Preheat oven to 350 degrees. Rinse kale, drain and pat dry with paper towel. Be sure it's completely dry. Place in a large bowl and drizzle oil over it. Sprinkle with salt and toss to coat well. Place in a single layer on three cookie sheets. Bake at 350 degrees for 15 minutes, watching closely to prevent burning. Cool completely before serving.

These are extremely healthy and very tasty!

Sharon Fox

PARMESAN CRISPS

1/2 cup fresh Parmesan cheese
1/4 tsp. fresh cracked black pepper

Preheat oven to 400 degrees. Line a baking sheet with parchment paper. Spoon the cheese by tablespoonfuls about 2 inches apart. Spread each mound to about 2-inch diameter. Sprinkle with cracked black pepper. Bake 6-8 minutes or until golden and crisp. Cool completely on the baking sheet. Remove from sheet with a thin spatula.
Great party appetizer, or serve with a nice salad.

GLUTEN-FREE GUACAMOLE

2 medium avocados, diced
1/4 tsp. minced garlic
1/4 tsp. finely diced jalapeno
1/4 cup chopped tomatoes (seeded)
1 tsp. chopped onion
salt
2 tsp. fresh lime juice
2 tsp. chopped fresh cilantro

Mash the avocado, garlic, and jalapeno with a wooden spoon until the avocado is creamy but still chunky. Add the tomato, onion, and salt. Stir together to combine. Add the lime juice and cilantro. Stir to combine and taste. Serve with your favorite gluten-free chips or crackers.
Makes 2 cups.

LEMON FRUIT DIP

1/4 cup sugar, divided
1 large egg
2 1/2 Tbsp. fresh lemon juice
1/4 cup water
1 1/2 tsp. cornstarch
1/2 tsp. vanilla extract
1 1/2 cups frozen whipped topping, thawed

Combine 2 Tbsp. sugar, egg, and lemon juice in a small bowl. Whisk together to combine. Combine the remaining 2 Tbsp, sugar, and water in a small saucepan. Bring to a boil and cook 30 seconds, stirring constantly until thickened. Remove from heat and pour in the beaten egg mixture stirring constantly. Cook over medium heat for 2 minutes until thick, stirring constantly. Remove from heat and stir in the vanilla. Cool completely. Be sure the is no warmth left. Gently fold into the whipped topping. Serve with fresh pineapple, strawberries, or any fresh fruit slices.
Makes about 14 servings about 2 Tbsp. each.

SWEET N SPICY PECANS

1/3 cup sugar
3/4 tsp. cayenne
1/2 tsp. salt
1/2 tsp. ground coriander
1/4 tsp. ground cinnamon
1/8 tsp. ground allspice
1 large egg white
2 tsp. vegetable oil
2 cups pecan halves

In a bowl, mix together sugar and all the spices. Whisk in the egg white and vegetable oil. Mix well. Stir in the pecan halves. Spread the nuts in a single layer on a oiled non-stick 10x15-inch baking sheet. Bake at 300 degrees, stirring occasionally, for 20-25 minutes. Allow to cool about 5 minutes. Loosen from pan and cool completely. Store in an airtight container for up to 2 weeks. Serve at your next party!
Makes 2 cups.

Sharon Fox

COTTAGE CHEESE FRUIT DELIGHT

1 lb. cottage cheese
3 oz. jell-o powder mix
1 cup Cool Whip
4 oz. crushed pineapple, drained

Mix together in order given. Chill for 2 hours and enjoy! Makes 10 servings.

NOTES

NOTES

Chapter 20

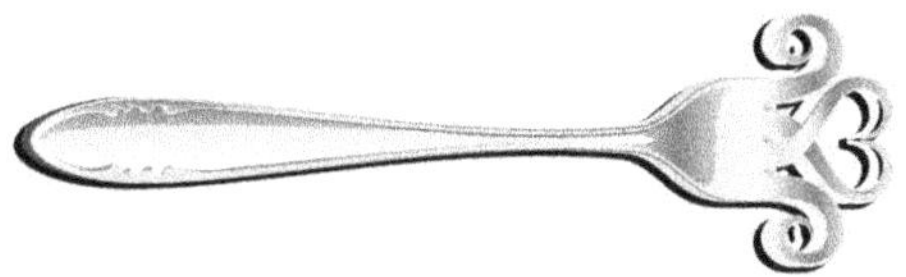

~SOUPS AND SIDES~

LOBSTER BISQUE

4 Tbsp. butter
2 Tbsp. scallions, finely diced
1 stalk celery with leaves, finely diced
4 Tbsp. gluten-free sweet rice flour
2 cups PLUS 2 Tbsp. half and half
1 Tbsp. tomato paste
2 tsp. paprika
1 tsp. Old Bay seasoning
1/8 tsp. cayenne (or to taste)
1/2 tsp. sugar
10 oz. cooked lobster meat, chopped (blot dry)
2-3 Tbsp. sherry
salt and pepper to taste

In a medium size heavy saucepan, melt butter over medium-low heat. Stir in the celery and scallions and cook until they begin to soften, about 3 minutes. Whisk in the rice flour and blend well. Cook about 3 more minute, stirring frequently. Slowly stir in the half and half until well combined. Add the tomato paste. Cook and stir over medium-low heat until it begins to thicken, about 3-5 minutes. Stir in paprika, Old Bay seasoning, cayenne, sugar, and sherry. Stir to combine and add lobster meat. Season with salt and pepper and simmer for about 5 minutes to heat through. Do not allow it to boil or it will curdle. Serve hot as is, or blend in a blender to make into a cream soup. Serve hot.. Makes 4 servings.

BEEF BURGUNDY STEW

2lbs. beef stew meat or sirloin, cut in 1-inch cubes
2 Tbsp. butter
2 Tbsp. olive oil
1 yellow onion, cut in 1-inch pieces
4 Tbsp. sweet rice flour
1 1/4 cups gluten-free beef broth
1 1/4 cups red wine
1 tsp. dried marjoram
1 tsp. dried thyme
1/4 tsp. cracked black pepper
8 oz. button mushrooms, wiped clean
8 oz. fresh pearl onions, peeled

Preheat your oven to 300 degrees. Put butter and olive oil in Dutch oven over medium heat. When it gets hot, add meat and cook until browned on all sides. Remove meat from pan and set aside. Add onions to pan and cook for about 5 minutes, stirring until they begin to brown. Turn off the heat and sprinkle in the rice flour. Stir to combine. Slowly whisk in 1/2 cup of the beef broth.

Turn heat back on to medium and cook mixture becomes smooth and slightly thickened. Add the remaining broth and red wine. Stir to combine everything well. Add salt, pepper, marjoram, and thyme. Stir, cover and place in oven for 2 hours. After the 2 hours add the mushrooms and pearl onions. Cover and return to oven 30 minutes more. Cool slightly and serve with your favorite toasted gluten-free bread. Makes 4 hearty servings.

CHICKEN GUMBO

1/2 cup light olive oil or canola oil
1/2 cup gluten-free rice flour
1 1/2 cups chopped onions
1/2 cup chopped celery
1/2 cup chopped bell pepper
1/2 cup sliced green onions
1 can diced tomatoes OR 1 lb. fresh tomatoes, diced
2 cloves garlic, minced
10 oz. pkg. frozen sliced okra
5 cups gluten-free low sodium chicken stock
1 lb. gluten-free smoked sausage, sliced
1 lb. cooked chicken breast, shredded
1 tsp. salt
1/2 tsp. thyme
3 bay leaves (remove before serving)
1/2 tsp. cayenne pepper
4 cups freshly cooked rice
Tabasco sauce
Fresh parsley for garnish, optional

Make a roux by combining the oil and flour in a heavy stockpot. Whisk constantly over medium heat until it turns to a deep caramel color. Remove from heat as soon as this color is reached. Add onions, celery, bell pepper, and green onions. Return to medium heat. Cook and stir until veggies are tender, about 3-5 minutes. In a heavy skillet over medium heat, cook and stir the okra just until it begins to release the stringy rope-like natural juice. This should take about 10-15 minutes.

Add the okra, chicken stock, sausage, chicken, tomatoes, and garlic to the stockpot. Simmer for about 30-35 minutes. To serve, put about 1/2 cup of rice into bowls and add the gumbo. Garnish with parsley and add a few drops of Tabasco. Makes about 8 servings.

NAVY BEAN AND CORNED BEEF SOUP

2 15 oz. cans navy or great northern beans, rinsed and drained
1 large onion, finely diced
2 stalks celery with leaves, finely diced
1 Tbsp. Italian flat-leaf parsley, minced
1 cup fresh spinach, chopped
2 cloves garlic, minced
4 cups gluten-free low sodium chicken stock
2 cups gluten-free corned beef, cubed
1 Tbsp. olive oil
1/2 tsp. dried thyme
salt and pepper to taste

In a medium size stockpot, heat olive oil over medium heat. Cook the onions, celery, garlic, and spinach for about 2 minutes, stirring until spinach wilts. Stir in the rinsed beans, chicken stock, corned beef, and thyme. Bring to a boil and then reduce heat to simmer for about 45 minutes, covered. Remove 2 cups of the soup and put it in a blender. Puree and return to soup pot.
If you don't have a blender, just mash the 2 cups of soup with a wooden spoon. The mashed beans serve as a natural thickener. Return the mashed portion back to the pot.
Season to taste with salt and pepper. Makes 6-8 servings.

***** This soup tastes even better if you make it the day before you want to serve it! The flavors have a chance to be enhanced.***

5 GLUTEN-FREE CREAM-O-VEGGIE SOUPS

3 1/2 cups gluten-free chicken broth
3 Tbsp. olive oil or butter
3 Tbsp. amaranth flour
1 clove garlic, minced
salt to taste
1 Tbsp. gluten-free onion powder
1 1/2 cups half and half OR light coconut milk
3 cups fresh vegetables
fresh cracked pepper

Steam your fresh veggies until just tender, do not over-cook. Set aside. Melt butter or heat olive oil in a large stockpot over medium heat. Whisk in the amaranth flour to make a paste. Add garlic and cook for 30 seconds to 1 minute, stirring constantly. Slowly add chicken broth, whisking constantly. Keep whisking and cooking until smooth and creamy. Add the steamed veggies, cream, and seasonings and stir until smooth. Remove from heat and allow to cool a bit. Pour into a blender (in batches) and blend until smooth. Re-heat over medium heat, do not boil. Serve.

The 5 Variations:

Fresh Cream of Asparagus Soup - Steam asparagus until tender. Add 1/2 tsp. nutmeg and 1 Tbsp. fresh lemon juice.

Fresh Cream of Broccoli Soup - Steam broccoli until tender. Add 1 Tbsp. fresh thyme OR 1/2 tsp. dried thyme.

Fresh Cream of Mushroom Soup - Chop Portobello mushrooms and saute them in 1 Tbsp. butter or olive oil until tender. Add 1/2 tsp. nutmeg and 1 Tbsp. dry sherry.

Fresh Cream of Potato Soup - Boil peeled cubed potatoes until tender. Cook 1/2 cup thinly sliced leeks or onions in 1 Tbsp. butter. Dice 1 strip of cooked bacon. Add 1/2 tsp. dried thyme

Fresh Cream of Tomato Soup - Peel tomatoes, remove seeds and chop flesh. Add 1 Tbsp. fresh basil, chopped or 1 tsp. dry basil and 1/4 tsp. dried oregano or 1/2 tsp. fresh oregano.

Sharon Fox

GARLIC PARMESAN MASHED RED POTATOES

2 1/2 lbs. red potatoes, unpeeled and quartered
3 cloves garlic, peeled and halved
2 Tbsp. butter
1/2 cup milk or organic coconut milk
1 tsp. salt
1/4 cup grated fresh Parmesan cheese

Put the potatoes and garlic in a large pot. Cover with water and bring to a boil. Reduce heat and simmer for 25 minutes, until potatoes are tender. Drain well. Put them back in pot. Mash with butter, milk, and salt. Stir in the cheese. Makes 6 servings.

SPICY CORN

10-12 ears of fresh corn, shucked
3/4 cup gluten-free vegetable or chicken broth, divided
2 Tbsp. olive oil
1 cup yellow onion, chopped
1 jalapeno pepper, seeded and diced
1-2 Tbsp. fresh lime juice
1 Tbsp. fresh basil, shredded
salt and pepper to taste

Cut the corn off the cob, you should have about 6 cups. In a blender, combine 1 cup of the corn kernels and 1/2 cup of the broth. Puree until smooth and set aside.

Heat oil in a large skillet over medium heat. Add the onion and a pinch of salt. Reduce heat to low and cook about 8 minutes, stirring occasionally. Add remaining corn and another pinch of salt and cook 3 minutes. Add the diced jalapeno pepper and pureed corn and bring to a simmer. Cook 2 minutes. Stir in the remaining broth, lime juice, and basil. Season with salt and pepper to taste. Simmer for a few more minutes until done, about 5-8 minutes. Makes 6 servings.

Sharon Fox

CARAMELIZED BUTERNUT SQUASH

2 medium butternut squash (4 or 5 lbs. total)
6-8 Tbsp. unsalted butter, melted and cooled (or canola oil)
1/4 cup light brown sugar
1 1/2 tsp. salt
1/2 tsp. black pepper

Preheat your oven to 400 degrees. Cut off the ends of squash and peel. Cut the squash in half lengthwise. Use a spoon to remove the seeds. Cut into 1 1/2-inch cubes and place on a cookie sheet sprayed with cooking spray. Pour the melted butter over cubed squash. Top with brown sugar, salt, and pepper. Toss to coat well. Roast in oven for 45- minutes to 1 hour, until squash is tender, caramelized, and glazed. Turn a few times during baking process to be sure it cooks evenly. Serve hot. Makes 6 servings.

LOW CARB LOADED CAULIFLOWER (BETTER THAN BAKED POTATOES!)

2 1/2 cups cooked cauliflower
1 cup low-fat sour cream
3/4 cup shredded cheddar cheese
3 green onions, chopped
3-6 slices bacon, crumbled (or turkey bacon)
salt and pepper to taste

Preheat your oven to 350 degrees. Chop the cooked cauliflower into chunks. In a medium size bowl, mix together the sour cream, half of the green onions, half of the cheese, half of the bacon, salt and pepper to taste. Stir in the cauliflower. Pour mixture into a greased medium size baking dish. Top with remaining cheese and bacon. Bake for 20 minutes. Right before serving, sprinkle with remaining green onions. Makes 3 servings.
Only 8g Carbs per serving!

Sharon Fox

ITALIAN BAKED ZUCCHINI

6 medium zucchini, thinly sliced
1 medium onion, chopped
1 large tomato, chopped
1 clove garlic, minced
8 oz. gluten-free tomato sauce
2 cups mozzarella , shredded
1 tsp. Italian seasoning
1 Tbsp. olive oil
1 tsp. garlic salt

In a large skillet, heat oil. Add zucchini, onion, garlic, and tomato. Cover and cook 10 minutes, until tender. Drain well. Stir in tomato sauce and seasonings. Spray a 9x13-inch baking dish with cooking spray. Place a layer of zucchini and top with cheese. Repeat until all is used up, ending with cheese. Bake uncovered at 350 degrees for 25 minutes or until cheese is browned. Top with some grated Parmesan or Romano when serving, if desired. Makes 8 servings.

PERFECT FLUFFY MICROWAVE RICE

1 cup rice (Basmati or Persian works best)
2 cups water
1/8 tsp. salt

Put the rice in a microwave safe bowl. Add the water and stir briefly. Add the salt and stir again. Cover with vented plastic wrap or loose cover. Microwave on high for 12 minutes. Allow to sit for 5 minutes. Dump into a strainer and rinse under cool water.

Place back in bowl and season to taste however you want. Heat on medium for 5 minutes or until hot enough for you. Makes 6 servings.

Sharon Fox

SPINACH-ARTICHOKE SMASHED POTATOES

1 lb. baby Yukon gold potatoes, quartered
14 oz. can artichoke hearts, drained
10 oz. pkg. frozen spinach, thawed
1/4 cup skim milk
1/4 cup sour cream
2 Tbsp. margarine
2 Tbsp. grated Parmesan cheese
1 clove garlic, minced
salt and pepper

Put potatoes in a large pot and cover with water. Add a little salt. Bring to a boil and then reduce to simmer. Cook for 20 minutes or until tender. While potatoes are cooking, puree half of the artichoke hearts in a food processor. Set aside.

Roughly chop remaining artichoke hearts, set aside. Squeeze water from spinach and season with a little salt and pepper, set aside. Drain potatoes and return to pot. Add the pureed artichokes, margarine, Parmesan cheese, sour cream, milk, and garlic. Mix with an electric mixer until creamy. Fold in the chopped artichokes and spinach. Season to taste. Makes 4 servings.

LEMON HONEY-MUSTARD CARROTS

1 lb. baby carrots
1 tsp. Dijon mustard
1 tsp. extra virgin olive oil
1 1/2 tsp. honey
1 tsp. lemon juice

Steam the carrots until done.
Whisk together remaining ingredients in a small bowl. Drizzle over cooked carrots. Serve. Makes 4 servings.

NOTES

Chapter 21

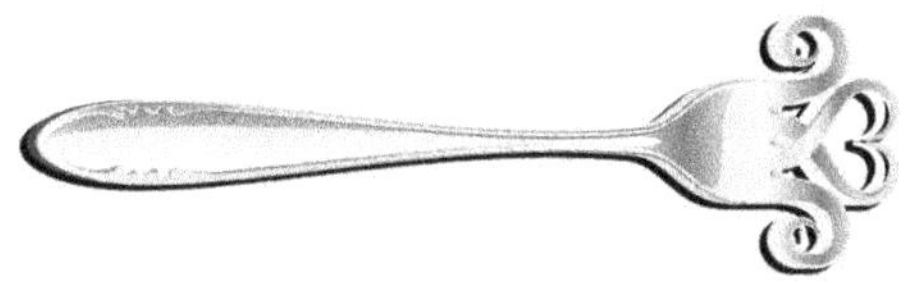

~MAIN DISHES~

ITALIAN MEATBALLS

1 lb. lean ground beef
1/2 lb. ground pork
1 large egg, slightly beaten
1/2 cup grated Parmesan cheese
1/3 cup instant potato flakes OR gluten-free bread crumbs
1-2 Tbsp. fresh garlic, minced
2 tsp. salt
1 tsp. black pepper
1/3 cup milk or milk substitute (use up to 1/2 cup if needed)
1/2 tsp. dried oregano
1/4 cup fresh parsley, chopped (or 2 Tbsp. dried parsley)
your favorite gluten-free spaghetti sauce

In a large bowl, combine all ingredients except the spaghetti sauce. Mix well until combined but don't over work the meat the meatballs will be tough. Shape into meatballs and place on a baking sheet OR you may drop them in your favorite sauce and allow them to simmer 20 minutes without stirring. Allow to simmer 20-25 more minutes, until done.

If you decide to bake them, preheat oven to 350 degrees and bake for 25 minutes. Serve with your favorite gluten-free pasta and sauce. Serves 6

Sharon Fox

CHICKEN WITH PEACH-CUCUMBER SALSA

1/2 cup chopped cucumber
1/3 cup peach preserves
1 Tbsp. fresh mint leaves, chopped
1/4 tsp. salt
2 Tbsp. red onion, chopped
1 fresh peach (or nectarine), chopped (about 3/4 cup)
4 boneless, skinless chicken breasts
salt and cracked black pepper

Spray grill rack or grill pan, if cooking indoors, with non-stick cooking spray. Heat to medium heat. Season chicken with salt and pepper on both sides with salt and pepper.
In a small bowl, combine the cucumber, 2 Tbsp. of the preserves, mint leaves, salt, onion, and peach. Set aside.
Cook the chicken for 10-15 minutes, turning 2-3 times during cooking and brushing with the remaining preserves. Cook until the juices of the chicken run clear. Serve with the salsa. Makes 4 servings.

ASIAN CHICKEN STIR FRY

1/4 cup gluten-free chicken broth
1 Tbsp. cornstarch
1 Tbsp. sugar
2 Tbsp. gluten-free soy sauce
1 Tbsp. apple cider vinegar
1/4 tsp. cayenne pepper
2 Tbsp. vegetable oil
1 lb. boneless, skinless chicken cut in cubes or strips
1 small onion, cut into 1/2-inch wedges
2 cloves garlic, minced
1 tsp. ginger root, grated
1 1/2 cups fresh hericot verts (baby green beans)
1 medium red bell pepper, cut into 1-inch pieces
2 Tbsp. water
1 cup fresh pineapple, cut in 1-inch cubes
1/3 cup gluten-free dry-roasted peanuts
*cooked rice or gluten-free pasta, for serving

Mix the first six ingredients in a small bowl to make the sauce. Set aside. In a wok or nonstick skillet, heat 1 Tbsp. of the oil over high heat until it shimmers. Add the chicken, onion, garlic, and ginger root. Cook for about 1 minute without stirring. Stir fry for about 3 minutes until chicken is cooked through. Put the chicken mixture in a bowl and set aside. Add the remaining 1 Tbsp. of oil to the wok or skillet. heat for about 1 minute, add the green beans and bell pepper. Stir fry for 2 minutes. Add the water, stir, and cover for 1-2 minutes. Stir and add the chicken mixture back to the pan. Whisk the sauce again to combine ingredients and pour over chicken and vegetables. Stir to coat and cook until thickened, about 1 minute. Stir in the pineapple and nuts. Serve immediately with cooked rice or gluten-free pasta. Makes 4 servings.

BEEFY SPUDS

2 large baking potatoes
1/4 cup sour cream
1/2 lb. 80% lean ground beef
1/2 tsp. salt
1/4 tsp. pepper
1 cup frozen corn kernels
8 oz. can tomato sauce
2 green onions, sliced
1 Roma tomato, chopped
chives, thinly sliced

Bake your potatoes until tender. Let stand about 5 minutes until cool enough to handle. Cut them in half lengthwise. Scoop out pulp from potatoes, leaving about 1/4-inch border inside each potato half. Put the pulp in a medium bowl. Mash potatoes with sour cream, set aside.

In a skillet over medium-high heat, cook beef, salt, and pepper until beef is done and crumbly. Drain off fat. Stir in corn, tomato sauce, diced tomato, and onions. Cook 3-4 minutes, stirring frequently until hot and bubbly. Spoon the beef mixture into potato shells. Top with 1/4th of the mashed potato mixture. Heat in microwave for about 5 minutes or in oven 350 degrees about 15 minutes until heated through. Top with chives just before serving. Makes 4 servings.

VEGETABLE SPANISH PAELLA

3/4 cup uncooked long-grain brown or white rice
2 cups water
1 lb. asparagus, cut into 1-inch pieces
3 cups fresh broccoli florets
2 tsp. olive oil
1 medium red bell pepper, chopped
2 small zucchini, chopped
1 medium onion, chopped
1/2 tsp. salt
1/2 tsp. saffron threads OR 1/4 tsp. ground turmeric
2 medium tomatoes, seeded and chopped
2 (15oz.) cans garbanzo beans, rinsed and drained
10 oz. box frozen sweet peas, thawed and drained
large lettuce leaves, if desired for serving

Cook your rice as directed on package, set aside and keep it warm. In a 2-quart saucepan, heat 1-inch of water to boiling. Add asparagus and broccoli, return to boiling. Cook for about 4-5 minutes until crisp-tender. Drain. Heat a 10-inch skillet over medium-high heat. Add asparagus, broccoli, bell pepper, zucchini, onion, salt, and saffron or turmeric. Cook about 5 minutes until onion is crisp-tender. Stir in the remaining ingredients except lettuce leaves. Line platter or individual serving plates with the lettuce leaves. Pour the paella on top of the lettuce and serve. Makes 6 servings.

Sharon Fox

BRINED TURKEY BREAST

9 cups water
3/4 cup salt
1/2 cup sugar
1 bone-in whole turkey breast, thawed (4-6 lbs.)
1 onion cut into 8 wedges
2 sprigs fresh rosemary
4 sprigs fresh thyme
3 bay leaves
6 Tbsp. butter or margarine, melted
1/4 cup gluten-free chicken broth or dry white wine

In a large stockpot, add water, salt, and sugar. Stir until salt and sugar are dissolved. Place the turkey breast into this brine liquid. Cover and refrigerate for at least 24 hours, but no longer than 24 hours.

Preheat oven to 325 degrees. Remove turkey breast from brine, rinse, and pat dry. Put the onion in the center of rack of a large shallow roasting pan. Top with rosemary, thyme, and bay leaves. Place turkey skin side up on top of herbs and onion.

In a small bowl, stir together the butter and broth. Soak a 16-inch square of cheesecloth in butter mixture. Cover the turkey with the soaked cheesecloth. Roast in preheated oven for 1 1/2 hours. Remove the cheesecloth. Pour the drippings, onion, and herbs into another pot to make gravy later if you want.. Turn the turkey breast skin side down and roast 30-60 minutes longer, until it's done (165 degrees). Makes 8 servings.

This is a wonderful way to do your turkey breast for holidays or anytime!

GLUTEN-FREE OVEN FRIED CHICKEN

1 Tbsp. butter or margarine
1 cup Bisquick gluten-free mix
1 tsp. seasoned salt
1 tsp. paprika
1/2 tsp. garlic powder
1/4 tsp. pepper
2 eggs, beaten
1 whole chicken, cut up

Preheat oven to 400 degrees. Melt butter in a 9x13-inch baking pan in oven. In a medium bowl, combine the baking mix, salt, paprika, garlic powder, and pepper. Place the eggs in a shallow dish and beat them.

Dip the chicken pieces into egg and then into dry mixture to coat. Place skin side down in heated baking dish. Bake for 35 minutes, turn chicken and bake about 15-20 minutes longer. Juices should run clear when done. Makes about 5 servings.

BALSAMIC BROWN SUGAR GLAZED HAM

6-8 lb fully cooked smoked, bone-in ham (spiral-cut works well)
1 cup brown sugar
2 Tbsp. gluten-free balsamic vinegar (or apple cider vinegar)
1/2 tsp. ground mustard
orange slices and Maraschino cherries, optional

Heat your oven to 325 degrees. Place the ham, fat side up on the rack of a shallow roasting pan. Cover loosely and bake 1 hour 15 minutes. About 20 minutes before ham is done, remove from oven and pour off drippings. Remove any skin from the ham.
In a bowl, combine the brown sugar, vinegar, and mustard. Stir until sugar is dissolved. Brush onto ham and bake 20 minutes longer. You may top with orange slices and cherries before the final 20 minute baking period if you wish. Makes 12 servings.

APRICOT BOURBON GLAZED HOLIDAY HAM

1/2 cup apricot preserves
2 tsp. ground ginger
1/4 cup bourbon or pineapple juice
3 Tbsp. brown sugar
6-8 lb. fully cooked smoked, bone-in ham

Combine preserves, ginger, bourbon or pineapple juice, and brown sugar. Stir to dissolve sugar and set aside.
Preheat oven to 325 degrees. Place the ham in a shallow roasting pan and score the ham into diamond-shaped cuts. Brush with about 3 Tbsp. of the glaze. Bake 45 minutes, uncovered. Brush the remaining glaze on the ham and bake another 45 minutes. Remove from oven and cover loosely with foil. Let stand about 15 minutes before serving. Makes 10 servings.

ROASTED PORK TENDERLOIN

1 pork tenderloin (1 to 1 1/4 lb.)
2 tsp. fresh rosemary leaves
1/2 tsp. salt
1/2 tsp. dried sage
1/4 tsp. fresh cracked black pepper
1 large sweet potato, cut into 1 1/2-inch pieces
2 firm pears, unpeeled and cut into 6 wedges
1 medium size sweet onion, cut into 6 wedges
1 Tbsp. olive oil

Heat your oven to 450 degrees. Spray a 10x15x1-inch baking sheet with cooking spray. Place the tenderloin on the sheet. In a small bowl, combine rosemary, sage, salt, and pepper. Rub half of this mixture onto the pork.

In a medium bowl, toss the sweet potato, pears, and onion with oil until coated well. Sprinkle the remaining seasoning mixture over the veggies and toss to coat. Arrange the seasoned vegetables around pork. Bake for 30-35 minutes, until pork is done. Stir veggies occasionally to allow even cooking. Remove from oven and cover with foil. Let sit 5 minutes and then cut into half-inch slices. Serve. Makes 4 servings.

ITALIAN LASAGNA

1 lb. gluten-free bulk Italian sausage of ground beef
(even better with half beef and half sausage)
1 medium onion, chopped
8 oz. pkg. fresh mushrooms, sliced
25 oz. jar gluten-free marinara or spaghetti sauce
15 oz. can gluten-free tomato sauce
1/2 cup water
1 1/2 tsp. dried basil
15 oz. gluten-free ricotta cheese
1/4 cup gluten-free Parmesan cheese
2 Tbsp. chopped fresh parsley
3 cups gluten free mozzarella cheese, shredded
12 uncooked gluten-free lasagna noodles

In a 4 quart pot, cook the meat, onions, and mushrooms until meat is no longer pink. Drain off fat. Stir in spaghetti sauce, tomato sauce, water, and basil.

In a medium bowl, mix the ricotta and Parmesan cheeses, and parsley. Heat oven to 350 degrees. In a 13x9-inch greased glass baking dish, spread 1 cup of the sauce. Layer with 4 of the uncooked noodles, half of the ricotta cheese mixture, and one-third of the sauce. Top with 1 cup of the mozzarella.

Repeat twice. Top with remaining mozzarella and sprinkle with additional parsley, if desired. Spray a sheet of foil with cooking spray and cover the lasagna. Bake 50 minutes, uncover and bake 10-15 minutes longer to brown the cheese. Let stand 10 minutes before cutting. makes 8 servings.

NOTES

Chapter 22

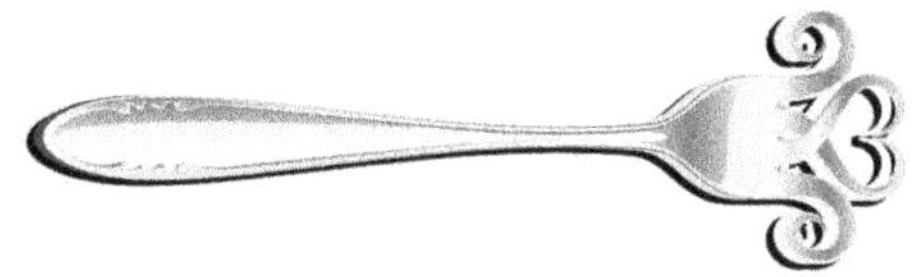

~GLUTEN-FREE DESSERTS~

SNICKERDOODLES

1/2 cup vegetable shortening
3/4 cup sugar
2 eggs
2 3/4 cups gluten-free baking mix
1 tsp. vanilla

Dipping Mixture:
3 Tbsp. sugar
2 tsp. cinnamon

Preheat your oven to350 degrees. Cream together the shortening and sugar. Beat in eggs, one at a time. Add vanilla. Stir in the gluten-free baking mix. Chill the dough for 1 hour to make it easier to handle.
Roll dough into 1-inch balls. Mix the sugar and cinnamon in a small bowl. Roll the cookie balls in the cinnamon mixture and place 2 inches apart on a greased baking sheet (or lined with parchment paper). Flatten each cookie with the bottom of a drinking glass that has been dipped in sugar/cinnamon mixture. Bake for 8-10 minutes. Cookies should be golden around the edges. Allow to cool on the cookie sheet for a few minutes before moving them to a cooling rack.
Keep cooled cookies in a plastic container or cookie jar. Makes 2 dozen cookies

CHOCOLATE CHIP PECAN COOKIES

3/4 cup butter, softened
1 1/2 cups brown sugar
1 egg
2 1/4 cups gluten-free baking flour
1 tsp. baking soda
1 tsp. baking powder
1 tsp. salt
1 cup chocolate chips
3/4 cup chopped pecans

Preheat your oven to 375 degrees. Line baking sheet with parchment paper. In a medium size mixing bowl, cream together the butter and sugar. Add the egg and mix well. Sift together the gluten-free flour, baking powder, baking soda, and salt. Slowly add to the creamed mixture. Stir in the chocolate chips and nuts.

Drop by teaspoonfuls onto prepared cookie sheet. Bake about 8 minutes, until slightly browned. Let cool on cookie sheet for 5 minutes before removing to cooling rack. Makes about 20 cookies.

CARAMEL DELIGHTS COOKIES

1 cup butter, softened
1/2 cup sugar
2 cups all purpose gluten-free flour
1 tsp. baking powder
1/2 tsp. salt
1/2 tsp. vanilla extract
1 to 2 Tbsp. milk

Cream together the butter and sugar. Sift together the dry ingredients and slowly add to the creamed mixture. Add vanilla and only enough milk to make dough come together. Chill overnight or at least 6 hours.
Preheat your oven to 350 degrees. Scoop out tablespoons of dough and flatten to 1/4-inch thickness. You can put a hole in the middle if you want them to be like the Girl Scout cookies!
Place on parchment lined cookie sheet and bake 12-15 minutes or until bottoms are brown and cookies are set. You may need to bake them up to 25 minutes, depending on your oven. Cool on baking sheet for 5 minutes before removing to cooling rack. Cool completely as you make the topping.

Topping:

3 cups shredded coconut
12 oz. bag of Kraft Caramels
3 Tbsp. milk
8 oz. Ghirardelli bittersweet chocolate chips
Preheat oven to 300 degrees. Spread coconut out on cookie sheet and bake until toasted, stirring occasionally. Cool completely on cookie sheet. While coconut is toasting, melt the chocolate in a small bowl in microwave.
Dip the base of each cookie in melted chocolate and place on wax paper to dry. Set extra chocolate aside. Unwrap caramels

and place in a microwave safe bowl with the milk. Microwave to melt, stirring in the milk to make creamy, 3-4 minutes. Fold in the toasted coconut. Spread 2-3 teaspoons onto each cookie. If caramel begins to firm up, just heat it in the microwave a few seconds to soften. Once all cookies are topped, drizzle the chocolate over them. (Melt chocolate again if it's already set up.) Makes 3 1/2 to 4 dozen cookies. These are wonderful for holidays or when you just want a special treat.

THE BEST GLUTEN-FREE BROWNIES EVER

2 1/2 cups powdered sugar
2 cups almond flour
2/3 cup unsweetened cocoa powder
1/8 tsp. salt
4 egg whites
2 tsp. pure vanilla extract

Line an 8x8-inch baking pan with parchment paper so there is about 3 inches overlaying all 4 sides. Preheat oven to 350 degrees. In a large bowl, combine the first 4 ingredients. Add egg whites and vanilla. Fold to combine all ingredients well. Pour batter into prepared baking pan.
Bake for 40 minutes. Remove from oven and *IMMEDIATELY* remove brownies from pan onto a cooling rack. Cool completely before cutting into squares.

Sharon Fox

ROCKY ROAD S'MORES BARS

1/2 cup brown rice flour
2 1/2 Tbsp. potato starch
1 Tbsp. plus 3/4 tsp. tapioca flour
1/4 tsp. xanthan gum
3 Tbsp. almond flour
3/4 cup gluten-free graham cracker crumbs
1/2 cup light brown sugar
1 stick cold unsalted butter, cut into chunks
1 large egg, slightly beaten

Topping:
3/4 cup semi-sweet chocolate chips
3/4 milk chocolate chips
2 Tbsp. heavy cream
1 cup gluten-free mini marshmallows
1/2 cup chopped walnuts

Preheat your oven to 350 degrees. Line the bottom and sides of a 9x13-inch baking pan with foil, leaving 2-3 inches of overhang on all sides. In a medium size bowl, sift together brown rice flour, potato starch, tapioca flour, and xanthan gum. Whisk in the almond flour.

In the large bowl of a food processor, combine the flour mixture, graham cracker crumbs, and brown sugar. Pulse to mix. Add butter and continue to pulse until mixture resembles cornmeal. Add egg and pulse just enough to mix. Press the dough evenly into the bottom of prepared pan and smooth the top. Bake until firm to the touch, about 20-25 minutes.

Meanwhile prepare topping. Coarsely chop 1/4 cup of the semi-sweet chocolate chips and 1/4 cup of the milk chocolate chips. In a saucepan over low heat, warm the cream until simmering. Add the chocolate chips, stirring until completely melted. Remove from heat and set aside. As soon as crust comes out of oven, sprinkle remaining chocolate chips, marshmallows, and walnuts over crust. Press down lightly with fingers. Drizzle the melted chocolate over the top and return the pan to oven. Bake until marshmallows puff up and begin to brown, about 7 minutes or so. Cool in baking pan on wire rack. If necessary, refrigerate until topping is firm, 1-2 hours. Lift out of pan, using the overhang as handles. Cut into 20 bars. Store in airtight container up to 5 days.

PERFECT GLUTEN-FREE VEGAN PIE CRUST

1 cup gluten-free all purpose baking mix
3/4 tsp. Xanthan gum
1 tsp. sugar
2 Tbsp. very cold butter (dairy or non-dairy)
3 Tbsp. organic shortening, very cold
2 tsp. Vodka (or water) chilled - adds flakiness!
8 tsp. cold water

Place butter, shortening, water, vodka, and a large mixing bowl into the freezer for 15 minutes to chill everything. This is very important for a flaky.

In a food processor, combine the flour, xanthan gum, and sugar. Process for 10 seconds to combine. While motor is running, add the butter and shortening until mixture is crumbly. Do not over process.

Pour the dough in your chilled bowl. Add the liquid ingredients 1-2 teaspoons at a time. Stir until dough starts to form. You may not need all of the liquid, so be sure to add just a little at a time. Place the dough into a glass pie plate and press with your fingertips to cover bottom and sides of entire pan. Flute edges as you like. Makes 1 9-inch pie. Fill pie crust and bake 20-50 minutes, according to your pie recipe!

GLUTEN-FREE GRAHAM CRACKER CRUST

2 cups crushed gluten-free graham crackers
1 stick butter, softened
2 Tbsp. sugar
1/4 tsp. nutmeg

Place the graham cracker crumbs in a bowl and add soft butter, sugar, and nutmeg. Use your fingers to combine all ingredients. Pour the mixture into a 9-inch pie plate or spring-form pan and press evenly to desired shape and thickness. Bake at 375 degrees for about 8 minutes. For a chilled crust, just chill the crust in refrigerator until firm. Makes 1 9-inch pie crust.

FROZEN KEY LIME PIE

1 recipe gluten-free graham pie crust
14 oz. can sweetened condensed milk (fat-free works well too!)
3 large egg yolks
1/2 cup fresh key lime juice
2 tsp. lime zest
1 cup Cool Whip
8 thin slices of lime, for garnish

Preheat oven to 350 degrees. Prepare one gluten-free 9-inch graham cracker pie crust. Bake crust for 5 minutes.
Combine the sweetened condensed milk, egg yolks, lime juice, and lime zest in a medium size bowl. Beat until smooth and thick. Pour into prepared crust and smooth evenly. Bake for 10 minutes, until crust begins to brown. Cool completely on a rack and then chill for 3-4 hours. Garnish with a dollop of Cool Whip and a thin slice of lime. Makes 8 servings.

CREAMY STRAWBERRY PIE

3 8oz. cartons strawberry yogurt
3 Tbsp. sugar
8 oz. Cool Whip
1 tsp. vanilla extract
2 cups sliced strawberries
1 9-inch gluten-free graham cracker crust

Pour strawberry yogurt into a medium mixing bowl. Stir in sugar until dissolved. Add vanilla and mix well. Fold in Cool Whip and then sliced berries. Mix well. Pour into pie crust and smooth. Place in freezer until frozen. Allow to thaw 10 minutes before serving. 6-8 servings.

APPLE CRUMB PIE

1 9-inch gluten-free pie crust
7 Granny Smith apples peeled, cored, and thinly sliced
1/2 cup sugar
1 tsp. cinnamon
1/4 tsp. nutmeg
1/4 tsp. salt

Place crust in a 9-inch pie plate that has been sprayed with cooking spray. Prick the bottom with a fork to allow air to escape.
In a large bowl, combine apples, sugar, cinnamon, nutmeg, and salt. Set aside and allow it to make its own natural juices.

Crumble Topping:

3/4 cup light brown sugar
3/4 cup gluten-free flour
1/2 tsp. nutmeg
1/3 cup butter, chilled

In a small bowl combine the brown sugar, flour, and nutmeg. Cut in the cold butter with a fork until crumbly.

Preheat oven to 400 degrees. Spoon apple filling into pie crust, pouring all the natural juices over the top. Sprinkle all of the crumble topping over the entire pie. Use foil to cover the edges of pie so it won't burn. Bake at 375 degrees for about 35-40 minutes, or until topping is golden brown. Allow it to cool at least 1 hour before serving.

BASIC GLUTEN-FREE YELLOW CAKE

1 1/2 cups white rice flour
3/4 cup tapioca flour
1 tsp. salt
1 tsp. baking powder
1 tsp. xanthan gum
4 eggs
1 1/4 cups sugar
2/3 cup mayonnaise
1 cup milk
2 tsp. vanilla extract

Preheat your oven to 350 degrees. Grease and flour two 8-inch cake pans. Mix the rice flour, tapioca flour, salt, baking soda, baking powder, and xanthan gum together and set aside.
Beat the eggs, sugar, and mayonnaise until fluffy. Add the flour mixture, milk, and vanilla and beat well. Pour into prepared cake pans and bake for 25 minutes, until golden brown and done. Insert a toothpick in the center to check for doneness. Let cool completely before frosting with your favorite icing or whipped topping. Great for birthday cake! Makes 24 servings.

SIMPLE GLUTEN-FREE CHOCOLATE CAKE

1 1/2 cups gluten-free flour blend
1/2 cup cocoa powder
1 cup sugar
1/2 tsp. salt
2 tsp. baking soda
3/4 tsp. xanthan gum
5 Tbsp. vegetable oil
1 Tbsp. vinegar
1 tsp. vanilla extract
1 egg
1 cup water

Mix all DRY ingredients together in one bowl. Mix all WET ingredients together in a separate bowl. Pour the liquid ingredients into the dry ingredients and mix well. Bake in a greased and floured 9-inch square pan in a 350 degree oven for 30-35 minutes, until a toothpick inserted in center comes out clean. Make the delicious chocolate syrup (ganache) to pour over the top!

Chocolate Ganache :

2/3 cup heavy cream
1 Tbsp. butter
8 oz. dark chocolate, chopped
2 tsp. vanilla extract

Heat cream and butter over low heat just until it simmers and butter melts. Turn off heat and add the chocolate. Allow it to sit for just a minute until chocolate melts. Stir to smooth it out and add vanilla. Stir. Pour over cake, cupcakes, or ice cream!

NOTES

NOTES

~Gluten-Free Cooking Tips~

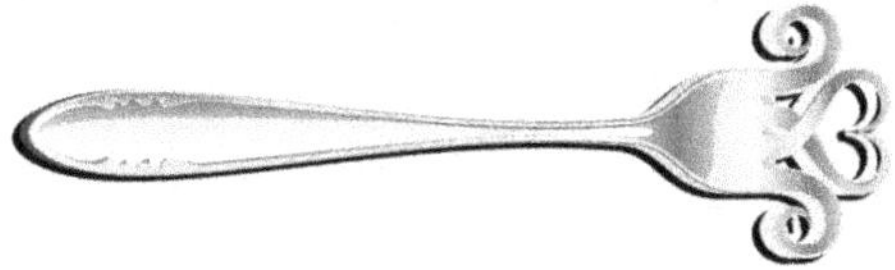

There are many tips and points to keep in mind when you're preparing new recipes for Celiac patients. It is so easy to pick up gluten from many items that you may not think would contain it. The two most important things I can tell you are:

1. Keep your work area clean! Be very sure that your work surfaces, utensils, and cookware are especially clean and free of any crumbs, dough, or any "stuck-on" items. Gluten can be carried from the utensils right into your food without your knowledge.
2. Always check labels of the products you're using in your recipes to insure that they are truly gluten-free. Manufacturers can change product information without notice. When in doubt, do not buy a product until you call or email the manufacturer for verification that it is gluten-free.

Finding the right foods and ingredients can be tricky, but not impossible. If you enjoy fresh fruits and vegetables, then you'll be glad to know that you're pretty safe, with a few exceptions. They are gluten-free. So don't hesitate to indulge in fresh berries, fruits, and vegetables bought in the produce section of your grocery store. There are a few items in the produce area that may contain gluten and you need to be careful to avoid those items. This will include jars of processed fruit and sauces, and pre-cut fruits and vegetables. Read the label carefully to be sure they are prepared in a gluten-free environment. Some stores cut the fruit up fresh in-store, but maybe in the bakery or meat market. Don't hesitate to ask. Better yet, just buy it whole and cut it up yourself. It's cheaper that way.

Chapter 23

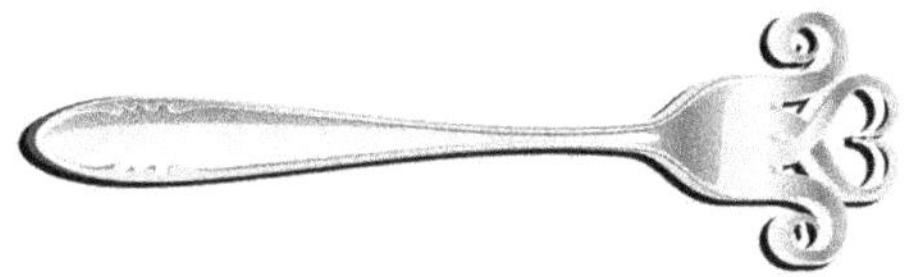

~GLUTEN-FREE SHOPPING~

I constantly stress to everyone I meet, always ask your doctor and/or nutritionist for tips and ideas for foods and products that may or may not be suitable for your own personal dietary needs.

This chapter will be very helpful to you in shopping for gluten-free groceries. There is no secret to finding the right products, you just need to know what to look for and what to avoid. Take note of this list, study it, and keep all these points in mind when shopping.

Canned and Frozen Fruits and Vegetables:

Many canned fruits and veggies are considered to be gluten-free, but some are not. The more ingredients listed on the label, the riskier the product. You may want to contact the manufacturer to see if the product is processed in a gluten-free environment or shared environment with other foods that contain gluten. This may seem like lot of work, but remember: your health is at stake.

Single ingredient frozen vegetables and fruits, like frozen carrots or corn, are generally safe but you need to read the label or contact the maker of the product to be certain. A few single ingredient frozen products are processed on the same lines as wheat products.

Some frozen mixed fruits and vegetables, like prepared side dishes with sauces, are not gluten-free. For this reason I stress reading labels.

Fish and Meats:

Usually fresh fish and meats are safe for the gluten-free diet, therefore fresh cut beef, pork, lamb, chicken, turkey, and fish can be considered a good product to buy. However, you must be aware of poultry and meats that have added ingredients that make them "ready-to-eat" or "ready-to-cook". These products may contain sauces or bread crumbs that could be a no-no to your diet. If the label doesn't actually say "gluten-free", it would be advisable to leave it in the store. Some chicken or turkey may even have a broth included that may not be safe, the label should specify this. This is one product you'll want to contact the manufacturer about the gluten content.

It's also a very good practice to avoid buying meat from meat-markets that do not have plastic wrapping on the meat. Fresh butcher shops often have "naked" meat in the cooler case for great presentation, but there is gluten all over the place! There are many meats or fish in the case that have bread crumbs or stuffing already in or on the meat. The use of fans blowing the meat can easily blow gluten all over other meats, without you even seeing it. Cross-contamination is highly found in meat cases like this. It's much safer to buy your meats pre-packaged.

Now let's take a look at hot dogs, ham, and other packaged meats. The USFDA (U.S. Food and Drug Administration) defines acceptable gluten-free as 20 parts per million. Very few of these products are labeled "gluten-free". You'll definitely need to contact the manufacturer for this information. Most hams usually will have an 800 number printed on the package for you to call. You can actually find gluten-free hot dogs and bacon pretty easily nowadays. Never assume a product is gluten-free if it isn't labeled so.

Sausage is a product that you really need to be careful purchasing. Many contain bread crumbs in their products as fillers, so check the label. Also, remember that gluten-free sausage could very well be packaged in a processing plant where gluten products are processed as well. You'll definitely need to call the manufacturer about this.

There are several gluten-free deli meats on the market. Hillshire Farms and Hormel are good brands that make a gluten-free line of meats. Boar's Head meat products are all gluten-free. However, the main thing to remember is the fact that deli shops can cross contaminate meats by slicing all meat on the same meat cutter. This practice can cause gluten to get on all of the meats. For this reason, pre-packaged deli meats are safer.

Dairy and Milk Products:

Most milk and dairy based products are gluten-free, but there are always a few exceptions. Plain milk, skim milk, and even heavy cream is naturally gluten-free. Where the problem may come in, is the flavorings that may be added, like strawberry or chocolate. You will definitely want to check the label to be sure. Another popular drink would be malted milk products. They are not safe because the malt is actually made from barley.

Yogurt is another product that is usually gluten-free, but you need to pay attention to the additives like cookies or granola, which do contain gluten. As you can see, reading your labels is very important.

The refrigerated dairy case carry many gluten-free products, such as tapioca pudding, eggs, butter, and margarine. You really want to check the ingredient labels on your margarine and shortening. Some milk substitutes are gluten-free and some are not. Soy milk and rice milk are both great gluten-free products to keep on hand. Please be careful about the "Rice Dream" rice milk found in the dry goods section- not the dairy case. It is processed with barley enzymes and is NOT totally gluten-free. Purchase your gluten-free dairy products straight from the dairy case to be on the safe side.

Cheeses and ice creams are popular gluten-free products. However, you really need to watch for "beer washed" cheeses which is becoming a new fad of cheese makers. Another caution for you to notice is the bleu cheeses. Some manufacturers use wheat as a catalyst when making bleu cheese. You'll need to contact the product manufacturer to be sure about their cheese. One last note to remember is to be wary of cheeses that are cut, sliced, and /or cubed in the store or deli. This is very common in stores where they make party trays. Cross contamination is the problem here. You'll never really know for sure what all they have cut on that machine or with that knife. Be safe and buy your cheese pre-packaged or in a block and cut it yourself. Save money and be safe!

As for ice cream, just like yogurt, be wary of products that contain cookies or cookie dough and other added ingredients that more than likely contain plenty of gluten. I think you should buy plain vanilla gluten-free ice cream and add your own gluten-free cookies to it. Breyer's and Hagen Dazs both make terrific gluten-free ice cream combinations. The label will say that this product is totally gluten-free, so read carefully. And of course you should know that ice cream sandwiches are off limits. That chocolate cookie sandwich is not a treat for you. There are several frozen fruit pops and one of my favorites is the Dove Ice Cream Miniatures...totally gluten-free!

Breads, Snacks, and Cereals:

You should definitely know by now that when it comes to bread, you must only choose from a variety of gluten-free items. There is a wide variety of frozen gluten-free bread available in grocery stores today. Just remember, you must avoid any bread containing wheat.

Baked snacks must only be purchased if the label states that it is gluten-free. There is a very large variety of gluten-free products on the market now. Several manufacturers are even making gluten-free potato chips, pretzels, bagels, and waffles. Read, read, read the labels. Some chips contain added ingredients for special flavorings like "cheese-flavored, barbecue-flavored, or sour cream-flavored". These additions come with plenty of gluten, so stick to plain flavors.

Cereals and pastas are readily available in nearly all grocery stores in a gluten-free variety. Go through you local store and spend some time checking them out. The main tip to remember is to always be sure the label says gluten-free. Choose pasta that is made from corn or rice. Some pastas are even made with quinoa and many other unusual gluten-free grains.

Pre-made and Pre-packaged Foods:

If you know me, then you already know how I feel about pre-made meals. I think we all should take the time to get in the kitchen and cook fresh foods. However, if you really must buy a frozen dinner, please make sure it's specifically marked "gluten-free". Believe it or not, you can actually find a few products on the shelf that say "just add water" and they are actually gluten-free. These are common in the Thai or ethnic section of the store. Pizza lovers can also find many gluten-free items. There are vegan pizzas and frozen snacks in the "natural" foods freezer section.

People are really surprised to find out that many canned soups contain gluten. This is because flour is used as a thickener, and flour contains gluten. But fear not, there are some gluten-free soups out there. Progresso is one of my favorite brands. They make a great gluten-free line of soups. There are many top of the line gourmet brands out there that make gluten-free soups, but you'll need to make that famous phone call to make sure. I'd actually suggest that you write down all your favorite food brands and list their 800 numbers. Keep the list on your refrigerator and call them up anytime you have a question. Here is another tip: when you call to verify your interest in their gluten-free products, ask them if they have any coupons available. These manufacturers are happy to send coupons for FREE products. All of the extreme coupon shoppers know exactly what I'm talking about. Make your phone call pay off! Every time!

Gluten-Free Dry and Baking Mixes:

I love the fact that gluten-free baking mixes have become very popular. There are so many people who really love baking, and Celiac Disease has not stopped them in the least. I want you to do some homework here. Stroll down the baking aisle in your favorite grocery store and take a look at all the gluten-free baking products that are now available. There are bread mixes, muffin mixes, pizza crust mixes, cookie mixes, cake mixes...you name it. There is no reason for you not to enjoy your meals in this century with all the items that are on the shelf just waiting for you to try them out. Just be sure that whatever you buy says "gluten-free". Since there are many people who enjoy cooking from scratch, you must know that yeast, baking powder, and baking soda are generally gluten-free. It's still safe to check the labels for any added ingredients that you may not be aware of. The same applies to cocoa, chocolate, and other flavorings.

Using Oils, Sauces, Spices, and Condiments:

Condiments can be extremely tricky if you aren't careful. Many dressings, sauces, and common condiments use flour or other gluten filled ingredients as thickeners. This is one group of products that you want to be very careful when using. Making the manufacturers phone calls will definitely be encouraged here. Once you know which products are safe, keep a list of them and keep those products on hand. Be sure to check the labels frequently because, as I stated before, manufacturers have been known to change their ingredients without notice to the consumer. Stay on your toes.

Finding gluten-free tomato sauces to go with your gluten-free pasta is not hard at all. There are many name brand companies that are making a line of gluten-free products. Heinz ketchup is considered gluten-free, as is French's yellow mustard, and Kikkoman Soy Sauce. Ask your doctor or nutritionist about vinegars. Apple cider vinegars are usually safe, but be cautious of grain vinegars as they do contain enough gluten to cause problems.

When using oils, most of them are considered gluten-free: olive oil, canola oil, and corn oil are great. Do not purchase "specialty oils". These are the ones you find gift-boxed for the chef in the family. They can contain many grains or spices that could trigger illness.

Fresh herbs purchased in your produce market are perfectly safe, and I suggest using fresh herbs whenever possible. If you prefer to use dried spices, McCormick single ingredient spices have been found safe by the FDA and considered gluten-free. If you must use mixed spices, purchase them individually and mix them yourself. It is wise to call McCormick once in awhile to ask about their spices being gluten-free and processed in a gluten-free atmosphere. Salt and pepper is also gluten-free, just don't purchase those fancy pants flavored salts. Stick to the basics. When cooking, less is more. Use basic ingredients and enjoy the freshness.

Coffee, Tea, and Other Beverages:

The most popular beverages made by Coca Cola and Pepsi Co. are considered to be gluten-free by the FDA. Fruit juices are also gluten-free as long as they are 100% real juice. Although some really sensitive Celiac patients have reported that pure orange juice can cause minor reactions. Other fruit drinks and punches may contain gluten, this is where you need to read your labels. Invest in a juicer and make your own fresh juice. Keep some berries in the freezer year-round for great fruit juice every day.

Unflavored coffees and teas are naturally gluten-free. However, flavored coffee drinks and herbal teas DO contain gluten. Look for gluten-free products in your local health food store. You can even find some online!

If you are a beer drinker, you really need to look for gluten-free beer. Naturally beer is made from barley, and this can really have a bad reaction on Celiac patients. Whisky and gin are not safe to drink either, as they are derived from gluten grains. Wine is usually a safe beverage unless you are very sensitive. Other safe alcoholic drinks would be rum, tequila, and gluten-free vodka- they are derived from potatoes or grapes. One last thing to remember about alcoholic beverages is to be sure the mixers you use for cocktails are gluten-free.

NOTES

NOTES

Chapter 24

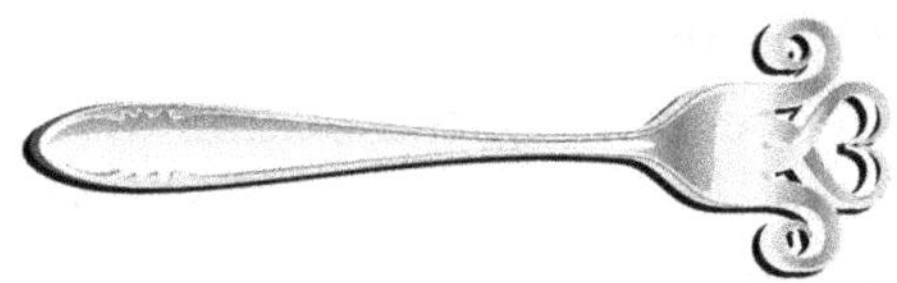

~CHILDHOOD OBESITY~

Overweight and obesity are the result of caloric imbalance. This means you are taking in more calories than you burn. This can be affected by genetic, behavioral, and environmental factors. CDC, 2012

Childhood obesity has both immediate and long-term effects on your child.

<u>Immediate Effects</u>:

- ❖ Children and teens who are obese are at higher risk of joint and bone problems, sleep apnea, social problems, psychological problems (stigmatization and low self-esteem).
- ❖ Obese teens are more likely to have pre-diabetes, their blood glucose levels indicate a high risk for developing diabetes.
- ❖ Obese children are more likely to have risk factors for cardiovascular disease (high cholesterol or high blood pressure).

Long-term Effects:

- ❖ Risk of many types of cancer: breast, colon, esophagus, kidney, pancreas, gall bladder, thyroid, ovary, cervix, prostate, and lymphoma.
- ❖ More likely to become obese adults which make them open targets for: heart disease, type 2 diabetes, stroke, cancers, and osteoarthritis.

Preventing Childhood Obesity should be one of the most important tasks of every parent in America. There are so many ways to help fight this disease and equip the children with habits and tools to get healthy and stay healthy.

Healthy habits, including healthy eating and regular physical activity, can lower the risk of our children becoming obese and developing related diseases.

The dietary and physical activity behaviors of children are influenced by social sector such as: families, communities, schools, physicians, churches, government agencies, the media, and entertainment industries. This is why we must be very careful about how we allow these sectors to mold our youngsters.

Schools play a critical role by establishing safe supportive policies, practices, and supporting healthy behaviors. Even though our children learn a lot about living healthy lifestyles in school, this is only one means of educating them.

As parents, we need to find new and creative ways to keep our children healthy and fit during their childhood years. Once they are in the habit of making healthy food choices and staying active, it won't be such a hard task when they are adults. it only takes 30 days to create a habit. Once you do something for 30 consecutive days, it becomes your daily ritual and not such a "job".

Tips For Parents:

- Limit convenience foods like, chips, cookies, and fast foods.
- Offer healthy meals and snacks that consist of fresh fruit and veggies, low-fat dairy products, whole grain breads and cereals, and lean sources of protein.
- Control portion sizes.
- Quench thirst with water instead of soda, juice, and sports drinks.
- Don't reward good grades or accomplishments with sweets.
- Involve the kids in grocery shopping, meal planning, and cooking.
- Discourage your child from eating in front of the TV, which causes you to eat more.
- Cut back on eating out, or order healthy options.
- Encourage physical activity. Family bike riding or walking is fun for all. Participate in team sports. Go bowling or challenge other families in weekly sporting activities.

Remember: Couch Potatoes breed Tater Tots! If you're lazy, you're going to encourage lazy children. Staying active is healthy for everyone, so get up and get busy!

Top 10 Best Snack for Kids:

1. Fruit - Kids require at least 1.5 cups of fruit per day. Why not make it fun? Use low-fat yogurt for dipping, or freeze some seedless grapes and serve them as a summer treat. Dried fruit is also a tasty treat.

2. Cereal - This is a great source of fiber, which is both healthy and filling. Don't offer the sugar sweetened "breakfast candy bowl" type of cereal for snacks. Instead, give them Cheerios, Honey Nut Cheerios, Life, or Kix.

These are easy to carry in a zip-lock bag while traveling, taking on short rides for errand trips, between meals, and even a TV snack.

3. Peanut Butter - Although high in fat, PB is a good source of fiber and protein. Spread some on graham crackers or with vegetable sticks with raisins.
4. Smoothies - Use handfuls of frozen fruit, like blueberries, pineapple, strawberries, and peaches along with some Greek yogurt, a banana, and believe it or not...a fistful of fresh spinach leaves! They will never taste the spinach or even see it for that matter. Give them all the nutrition you can in a smoothie!
5. Applesauce - Toddlers love applesauce, so give it to them. Kids like texture so add a few chopped apples, raisins, or their favorite chopped fruit. You can even freeze it in individual popsicle cups! Add some cinnamon for a great treat.
6. English Muffin Pizza - What kid will turn down pizza? Just split an English Muffin and top with pizza sauce and your favorite toppings. Make funny faces or designs and bake. What a great snack!
7. Meat Wraps - Get a tortilla and spread it with fat-free dressing. Layer it with lean deli meat and a slice of cheese. Roll up and slice into spirals. Kids love these when you allow them to put them together by themselves, with a little help from you.
8. Trail Mix - Allow your kids to create a bowl of fun by mixing all of their favorite snacks, like pretzels, Chex cereal, Craisins (dried cranberries), Cheerios, and nuts or dark chocolate chips.

9. Cheese - This is a good source of calcium. String cheese is very popular with kids. Also try cheese and wheat crackers or grilled cheese sandwiches.
10. Popcorn - This treat is packed with fiber and whole grains that can actually help lower your chances of developing diabetes or heart disease. Sprinkle with a little garlic powder or sweeten with just a touch of powdered sugar. Don't load it with butter and salt, you'll defeat the purpose.

Chapter 25

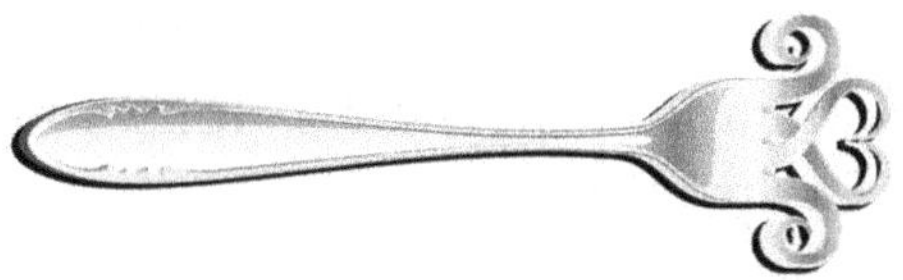

~HEALTHY TIPS~

Your body is your temple, and you need to take real good care of it to live a healthy, happy life. Don't ever compare your health or body to others. You are a beautiful, unique individual. Respect and love yourself enough to live your life to the fullest. Remember that you don't change your diet and exercise routine to be skinny, you do it to be healthy. Being skinny doesn't necessarily mean you're a picture of health. Get regular check-ups and follow your doctor's advice for your individual needs. Here are a few helpful tips to help you stay on track. It's not complicated, once you decide that your health is a top priority.

- ❖ Drink plenty of water. Over 60% of the human body is made up of water, therefore you need plenty of it to keep everything functioning properly. Water helps your body remove waste, carries oxygen, and transports nutrients through your body. Your body naturally loses water daily through perspiration, urine, and bowel movements, so it's very important to take in lots of pure water every day.
- ❖ Hang around healthy people. Surrounding yourself with others who have the same goals and ideas will encourage you to stay on track. Having buddies to walk, run,

workout, cook, eat, and talk with can be a big boost to your healthy lifestyle.

- Join classes or groups. This is a great way to meet others who have common interests. This is an important tip for those of you who are living in a new town or don't have friends who are into staying fit. Join some local dance classes, exercise groups, or a gym.
- Eat plenty of fresh fruit. Synthetic vitamins are not the same as consuming fresh food from nature. Oranges offer more health benefits than a vitamin C supplement. Indulge in these fresh fruits several times per day: Apples, avocado, apricots, grapefruit, cantaloupe, kiwi, guava, strawberries, watermelon, and papaya.
- Eat plenty of fresh vegetables. You really need to eat 5-9 servings of fruits and vegetables daily. The same rule applies to fresh veggies as fresh fruits. Natural foods are much better for you than supplements. Some key veggies include: Kidney beans, black beans, long beans, bean sprouts, mushrooms, carrots, sweet potatoes, and kale.
- Eat lots of colorful foods. This doesn't mean artificially colored foods! Naturally bright colored fruits and vegetables are usually high in antioxidants. Here is the color wheel of Health: White- mushrooms and bananas, Yellow- pineapple, mango, and bell pepper, Orange- oranges, papaya, and bell pepper, Red- apples, strawberries, tomatoes, red bell peppers, and watermelon, Green- avocado, guava, cucumbers, celery, bell peppers, kale, spinach, and lettuce, Purple/Blue- blueberries, prunes, eggplant, and dark cherries.
- Avoid binge foods. These are the foods that make to lose control when eating them. Some of the most common include: potato chips, donuts, and candy. These foods can cause an imbalance in blood sugar quickly.

Mental well-being is just as important as physical fitness. Staying focused and mentally energized can be complicated if you are not in a positive state of mind. Avoiding negativity is sometimes easier said than done if you are surrounding yourself with bad energy and people who do not have the same goals and thought process as you.

If you want to cleanse your mind, you really need to throw away all negative habits. I'm not bashing TV shows or telling you to get rid of your friends, but if they aren't pouring positivity into your spirit then you need to consider making some serious adjustments. Watch TV shows that encourage, educate, make you feel good, or make you laugh. These are what I call "feel good" shows. I avoid judge shows, baby-mama drama, and shows that get high ratings at the expense of the dignity of others. These shows will never do you any good.

As far as friends, you must choose them carefully. A true friend will encourage, inspire, assist, and enforce your decision to live a healthy life. Look at your circle of friends carefully and be sure they have these characteristics. If your circle of friends is draining you of all positivity and making you feel negative about your decision to live a better life, then I think it's time to get some new friends. You may end up encouraging them to make some great changes in their lives. Whatever the case may be, don't give up on your goals. You deserve to enjoy a long, healthy, happy life and it's up to you to take the necessary steps towards achieving it. Give it all you've got and reap the benefits of all your hard work.

Here are a few tips for creating a healthy spirit and mind.

❖ Get plenty of sleep. When you sleep well, you feel so much better the next day. Turn off the television during sleep hours because the sound of it actually interferes with sound sleep. Some people tend to think they sleep better with the TV on, but studies show that this is not true at all. As long as there is constant sound in your room, your brain is reacting to it. This is why you may feel exhausted half way through your day. Your brain really is tired! So do yourself a favor and get some sound sleep.

❖ Meditate often. Take some quiet time several times a day to just breathe deeply and clear your mind. This is a wonderful way to relieve stress. You may even want to buy or check out some books about different ways to meditate. It doesn't necessarily have to be a religious ritual. Meditation can actually give you that quality time you need to get away from everyone and everything. Try it for 15 minutes in the morning, mid-day, and night. You may want to start with 5 minutes each time until you get the hang of it. Just look at it as "me time". You deserve this time, so take it.

❖ Love yourself. List a few things about yourself that you are proud of and smile about each one. Repeat these things daily and add to the list often. The way you feel about yourself has a lot to do with the way you allow others to treat you. Remember that you deserve every good thing that life has to offer.

❖ Release all unhappy or negative thoughts. Deal with your issues as they arise, it's not good to hold these bad feeling inside. Release them through talking about them or writing them down and burying them. Once the feelings are released, don't allow yourself to harbor them again. If you find yourself holding on to the negativity, look in the mirror and tell yourself, "I will not allow this negativity to destroy my beautiful life. My positive life cannot live in the midst of negativity so I now release it from my being. I AM filled with positivity and prosperous energy from God." Inhale positive energy and exhale negativity. Do it often to stay in a positive mindset.

- ❖ Find your purpose. We all were born with at least one talent, gift, or activity that gives us "drive". Think about that one thing that you enjoy and also benefits others. Remember, your purpose is not just to satisfy yourself. Your purpose makes a difference in the lives of others and makes you feel absolutely amazing. Once you find out what your purpose is, do something every day to make it come alive. When you see how good you make others feel when you are doing what you were created to do, your life becomes more enjoyable. The joy that comes with your purpose cannot be bought. Find your purpose and live it!

No matter what your health condition may be at this point in time, remember that you still have a pulse. As long as you have that, there is always hope for a better tomorrow. You are worthy of living a happy life, filled with love and laughter. Treat yourself like you're living your dreams. If you want to lose weight, tone up, feel good, or just stay healthy - you can do it! There is nothing stopping you from being a better you, but you.

I pray that you find something in this book to turn your life around and put you on the road to an amazing new journey. There is so much to live for and so many more years to enjoy. If there is anything I can pass on to you, it would be to love yourself to the fullest and realize how important you are to this world. No matter how you got here, you're here on purpose and with purpose. I know that there are so many lives that can be changed, just because of you.

Keep living your best life and keep dreaming big dreams.

"Dreams are God's way of allowing you to see through His eyes."
- Sharon Fox

About the Author

Sharon Fox has been obsessed with food since she was a very small child. Over the past 36 years she has worked in the food industry on many different levels. Starting from the bottom and working her way up, she has been:

- cashier in a burger joint,
- cooked for large family occasions,
- worked as cake designer for a mega-market,
- studied food art
- catered private parties,
- designed wedding cakes,
- studied pharmacy and nutrition
- instructed healthy cooking classes for a large community in San Antonio, TX
- worked as a Private Chef,
- been a guest radio personality on several shows,
- hosted a TV show pilot
- and self published cookbooks!

Sharon's love and passion for food really shines through in every task she takes on.

"I feel that food brings everyone together. A good meal has no boundaries of race, gender, economic level, or religion."

After the release of ***COMFORT FOOD for the Mind, Body, and Soul,*** she received many requests for special diet recipes. Taking all of the questions and requests into consideration, ***HEALTHY FOOD for Diabetes, Celiac Disease and You!*** was written.

Websites and Contact Info:

http://www.goodcookin4u2.webs.com/
http://www.healthylivingshow.webs.com/
Facebook: https://www.facebook.com/sharonfoxauthor
Fan Page: https://www.facebook.com/icook4real
Twitter: http://www.twitter.com/ImSharonFox
Email: authorsharonfox@gmail.com

My Personal Journal

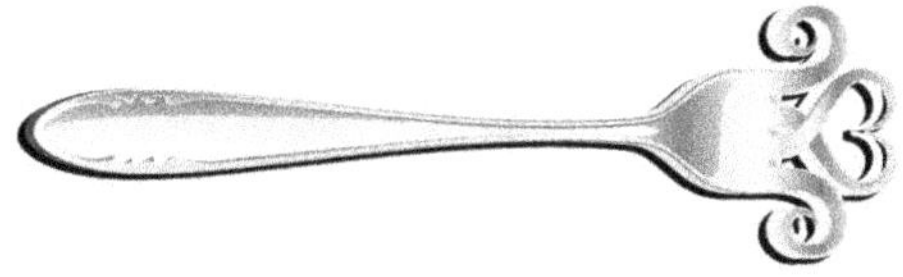

The following pages are strictly for your personal use. Jot down important information you may run across throughout your healthy journey! Set some goals, and keep track of your accomplishments.

I wish you many blessings and good health for the rest of your life!

~NEW FOODS TO TRY~

~IMPORTANT PHONE NUMBERS~

~MY SHORT TERM GOALS~
(3 to 6 months)

~MY LONG TERM GOALS~

(1 to 5 years)

~THINGS TO REMEMBER~
Life Lessons for Me

~IMPORTANT WEBSITES~

www.ingramcontent.com/pod-product-compliance
Lightning Source LLC
Chambersburg PA
CBHW060245100426
42742CB00011B/1650

* 9 7 8 0 6 1 5 7 2 0 1 5 9 *